Corticosteroids
in the
Treatment of Shock

Corticosteroids
in the
Treatment of Shock

Editors: WILLIAM SCHUMER, M.D.

Professor of Surgery, and
Chief, Surgical Service
University of Illinois College of Medicine
at VA West Side Hospital

LLOYD M. NYHUS, M.D.

Head of the Department of Surgery
University of Illinois College of Medicine

Published for the College of Medicine, Department of Surgery
by the
University of Illinois Press, Urbana, Chicago, London

A Symposium Conducted by the University of Illinois College of Medicine,
Department of Surgery
In Cooperation with the Division of University Extension
April 13, 1968, Illini Union, Chicago

Faculty

DENIS CAVANAGH, M.D.
Professor and Chairman
Department of Gynecology and Obstetrics
St. Louis University School of Medicine

CLARENCE D. DAVIS, M.D.
Professor of Obstetrics and Gynecology
Yale University College of Medicine

GORDON WATKINS DOUGLAS, M.D.
Professor of Obstetrics and Gynecology
New York University College of Medicine

WILLIAM DRUCKER, M.D.
Professor and Director
Department of Surgery
University of Toronto Faculty of Medicine

JACOB FINE, M.D.
Professor of Surgery Emeritus
Harvard Medical School

ROLF M. GUNNAR, M.D.
Professor of Medicine
Chief of University of Illinois Medical Division
    at Cook County Hospital

RICHARD C. LILLEHEI, M.D., Ph.D.
Professor of Surgery
University of Minnesota Medical School

JAMES C. MELBY, M.D.
Associate Professor of Medicine
Boston University School of Medicine

WILLIAM F. MENGERT, M.D.
Professor and Head
Department of Obstetrics and Gynecology
University of Illinois College of Medicine

LLOYD M. NYHUS, M.D.
Professor and Head
Department of Surgery
University of Illinois College of Medicine

WILLIAM SCHUMER, M.D.
Professor of Surgery
University of Illinois College of Medicine

WILLIAM C. SHOEMAKER, M.D.
Professor of Surgery
University of Illinois College of Medicine

WESLEY W. SPINK, M.D.
Regents Professor of Medicine
University of Minnesota Medical School

MAX HARRY WEIL, M.D., Ph.D.
Associate Professor of Medicine
University of Southern California
    School of Medicine

Preface

WILLIAM SCHUMER, M.D.

LLOYD M. NYHUS, M.D.

The subject of "Corticosteroids in the Treatment of Shock" allows us to touch all the important disciplines in the investigation of shock today. Our early morning sessions with Drs. Melby and Lillehei will cover the effect of corticoids on the pathophysiologic developments in shock. They will describe their physiologic studies of shock, specifically hemodynamic changes. Discussion of the pathologic changes in shock will be supported by the electron microscopic studies of Dr. Jacob Fine. Drs. Drucker and Schumer will review thoroughly the metabolic aspect. The clinical application of multidiscipline basic sciences will be presented by Drs. Weil, Spink, and Cavanagh. We have also included the investigative work of Dr. William C. Shoemaker and Dr. Rolf Gunnar. We felt that the inclusion of their studies would provide further background for the analysis of the efficacy of corticoids in shock. In these sessions, the knowledge acquired in the laboratory will merge with the pharmacologic studies, further developing the clinical treatment of patients.

The workshops offer the opportunity to expand on the morning lectures and stimulate discussion on controversial aspects from the panelists and the audience.

This symposium was designed to emphasize the fusion of basic and clinical sciences in the complex study of shock. Each discipline offers an explanation for the effect of shock, forming a collage of facts evolving into an intelligible picture of the etiology, pathogenesis, diagnosis, and treatment of shock.

Physiology   Biochemistry   Pathology   Pharmacology

Pathogenesis of Shock

Treatment of Shock

Contents

The Effects of Corticosteroids on Pathophysiology of the Shock Syndrome

Pathophysiology of Shock

JAMES C. MELBY, M.D.

LOCALIZATION AND MECHANISM OF EFFECT

Subcellular. Since 1960, little has been added to our knowledge of the action of corticosteroids. We know that their effect in protecting cells against noxious stimuli is nonspecific. Cells which have been exposed *in vitro* to such noxious stimuli as high concentrations of calcium in the extracellular medium, snake venom, toxic enzymes, acid hydrolases, and endotoxin can be protected by the presence of high concentrations of corticosteroids. We know also that the effect of corticosteroids is local, since they are effective against noxious substances only so long as they are unaltered and physically intact. The hormone must be present at the site of the inflammation. And finally, we know that the effectiveness of corticosteroids is proportionate to the amount of corticosteroids present at the inflammatory site. If one measures the volume of inflammatory tissue after a subcutaneous injection of an inflammatory agent, it can be seen that the amount of corticosteroid is inversely proportional to the volume of inflammatory reaction. Of course, the effect of corticosteroids in shock is a much

1

more complicated phenomenon and I will have more to say about that presently.

How do corticosteroids protect the cells? Steroids stabilize the plasma membrane, that is, the cellular and subcellular membranes. For example, if one adds steroids to a mixture of cells, the mechanical fragility of the cells decreases and the membrane stabilizes, even in red cells. Certain of the organelles within the cell also are stabilized. The most important of these organelles, which contain enzymes capable of perpetuating and intensifying the inflammatory reaction, is the lysosome, which has a lipid membrane. High concentrations of steroids will stabilize these bags of hydrolytic enzymes and protect them from rupturing after they have been exposed to noxious stimuli. Finally, there is stabilization of the membranous portion of the microcirculation. The rate and degree of diapedesis of both red and white cells are reduced in the presence of high concentrations of steroids.

Cellular. At the University of Minnesota in 1958, Dr. Spink and I[1] did some experiments that suggested the cell membrane might be stabilized by inhibition of the rise in glutamic oxalacetic transaminase after endotoxin injury. We gave 20 dogs lethal doses of *Escherichia coli* endotoxin. Ten of these dogs were also given large doses of cortisol by intravenous drip before and during the endotoxin challenge. We determined the serum transaminase levels during the six hours after injection of the endotoxin and found that these levels rose progressively in the animals that did not receive cortisol. In the dogs given large quantities of cortisol (about 30 mg/kg of body weight), the rise in serum transaminase levels was inhibited. Half the cortisol-treated dogs survived the critical 18-hour period of observation.

Endocrine. To determine the levels of cortisol present when the rise in transaminase was inhibited, the plasma cortisol levels were measured in the surviving animals and found to be 40 to 1,000 times higher than normal. These dogs had excellent cortisol-secreting ability in the face of a lethal dose of endotoxin. This study and subsequent studies by Weil[2] and others showed that the amount of cortisol required to inhibit transaminase elevation and allow survival of the experimental animal is several times that which the animal actually produces. For example, humans secrete between 10 and 30 mg of hydrocortisone daily under basal circumstances, and continuous corticotropin stimulation throughout a 24-hour period may increase the output to about 240 mg daily. A similar type of activity is observed in the dog, but the maximum secretory capacity of the dog's adrenal cortex is not sufficient to protect against the lethal effect of *E. coli* endotoxin.

Clinical Observations

For years it has been said that adrenal insufficiency was the cause of death because, on postmortem examination, bilateral adrenal cortical hemorrhage and acute adrenal insufficiency were found in shock patients who had had septicemia as a result of gram-negative or other microorganisms in the bloodstream. This problem of adrenal involvement was one of the first that I studied with Dr. Spink years ago, when he was investigating patients with the so-called Waterhouse-Friderichsen syndrome. In our early clinical studies of severe bacteremic shock, we grouped the patients as survivals or mortalities. Levels of plasma cortisol were very high in both groups, with a mean of 50 µg/100 cc in patients who recovered and 73 µg/100 cc in those who died. The mean under maximum stress usually does not exceed 65 µg/100 cc, and only rarely does the cortisol level achieved with ACTH stimulation exceed this level. Thus, in these patients with severe bacteremic shock, the cortisol levels were very high and neither in this group of patients nor in any groups studied subsequently have we ever encountered a patient in bacteremic shock who had low or reduced cortisol levels.

This observation has several implications. Dr. Spink and I[3] showed that these patients could respond to additional doses of ACTH and that actually their blood cortisol levels could rise still higher. There was thus no evidence in any patient in bacterial shock of a condition which would fit the description of the Waterhouse-Friderichsen syndrome of adrenal collapse. Although it seems strange today, we still see reports claiming acute adrenal insufficiency supervening in patients with bacterial shock, particularly meningococcal shock. It has never been demonstrated in any study that these patients are actually deficient in cortisol. They appear to have more than adequate amounts. On the other hand, there is evidence, which will be cited later, that patients in bacteremic shock may respond to huge doses of cortisol, but this represents a different situation.

As an example, I cite the case of a woman admitted on the Medical Service at the University Hospital in Boston, who had a *Pseudomonas* septicemia with profound shock and died after 24 hours of this shock state. Histologic examination of adrenal cortex revealed it to be relatively intact. Hemorrhage was limited to the medulla, as is true in most of the adrenal glands removed from patients with the Waterhouse-Friderichsen sydrome. It almost never completely destroys the cortex, as can be seen on examination of serial sections of the tissue. The patient had a plasma cortisol level of 120 µg/100 cc.

In our studies of patients who succumbed to meningococcemia with bilateral adrenal cortical hemorrhage, we found that all had plasma cortisol levels in excess of 100 µg/100 cc. At least as far as these observations go, I believe there is no evidence of acute adrenal insufficiency due to bacterial infections. Further, there is no evidence of acute adrenal insufficiency due to bilateral adrenal cortical hemorrhage, even if the hemorrhage is induced by dicoumarin or heparin; hence, whatever effect steroids have on this condition—and it appears to be considerable—it must be because the dosages are in a different range from those present physiologically, because there is plenty of cortisol present.

In both humans and dogs we have done a number of studies to determine the concentrations necessary to protect all the cells against an overwhelming endotoxemia. We found that, whether by the intramuscular, intravenous, or subcutaneous route, a maximum level of cortisol or any of its analogues can be obtained in one hour. It then begins to decline. The phosphate ester appears to give a higher blood level of the free corticosteroid than does the succinate ester.

Metabolism of Steroids

At the same time, by means of radioactive tracers, we studied the rate of metabolism of the steroids in animals, both in the normal state and the shock state. In general, our findings showed that in the normal state the rate of metabolism of corticosteroids is equal to their half-life in plasma. The half-life in plasma is much shorter in the normal state than in the shock state. The half-life of steroids is prolonged in the shock state and gives what amounts to a much higher level, probably because of hepatic decrease of enzymes of oxidation reduction in steroids. Hydrocortisone, or cortisol, has a half-life in tracer doses of about 80 minutes, prednisolone of about 200 minutes, methylprednisolone about 200, triamcinolone about 200 minutes, and dexamethasone about 300. Their half-life bears a strong relationship to the duration and intensity of their anti-inflammatory effects. Their half-life is noticeably prolonged in the shock state. One can decide on the necessity of repeating the dosage from knowledge of the half-life of the various steroid preparations. For example, repetition of cortisol dosage is required after 4 to 6 hours, methylprednisolone after 6 to 8 hours, and dexamethasone after 8 to 12 hours.

Dosage and Side-effects

We have used a range of steroid doses in the order of 500 to 1,000 mg of cortisone or pharmacologically equivalent doses of synthetic analogues. These figures were actually extrapolated from laboratory information initially, and it is largely due to the work of Lillehei, Weil, and Spink that we have these figures today. We have measured the levels after this kind of a dose, and they are astronomical in the human being. And this is apparently what is needed; because if all of the cell membranes of the organism are to be stabilized, a massive dose of corticosteroid is required.

From information derived from animal studies, we have developed a rationale and a procedure for the use of corticosteroids in medical emergencies—and we will probably get into more detail about this later in discussing endotoxin shock, acute tracheal broncheolitis, and a number of overwhelming toxemias and infections—and that procedure is to give steroids for a very brief period. It is our experience that a single injection of corticosteroid is often enough to restore the blood pressure in most animals and humans, and that the dose must be large. It must, in effect, be astronomical; that is, somewhere between 40 and 1,000 times that recommended as physiologic replacement. Dosage need not be tapered off. There is no prolonged suppression of pituitary-adrenal secretory activity after giving this kind of dose, and the side-effects are minimal in most instances.

There are, however, certain side-effects, including acute upper gastrointestinal ulcerations and intensification of diabetes mellitus, that are purported to occur with this dosage level of steroids. Intensification of diabetes mellitus can be dealt with if it is anticipated. We have not encountered acute upper gastrointestinal hemorrhage if the steroid is injected in a single bolus, or if the period of treatment is restricted to 24 hours.

REFERENCES

1. Melby, J. C., Bossenmeier, J. C., Egdahl, R. H., and Spink, W. W.: Suppression by Cortisol of Increased Serum-Transaminase Induced by Endotoxin, *Lancet* 1:441–444 (Feb. 28), 1959.

2. Weil, M. H.: Adrenocortical Steroid Therapy of Acute Hypotension, *Amer. Pract. Digest Treat.* 12:162–168 (March), 1961.

3. Melby, J. C., and Spink, W. W.: Comparative Studies on Adrenal Cortical Function and Cortisol Metabolism in Healthy Adults and in Patients with Shock Due to Infection, *J. Clin. Invest.* 37:1791–1798 (Dec.), 1958.

Hemodynamics

RICHARD C. LILLEHEI, M.D., Ph.D.

MICROCIRCULATORY CHANGES IN SHOCK

As an introduction to why we use steroids to treat the patient in
shock, I should mention briefly a few of the pathophysiological
mechanisms that seem to occur in shock.

In general, we feel that shock is characterized by initial vasoconstriction, or the ischemic type of microcirculation, and then,
in a shorter or longer time, a stagnant microcirculation; we will
hear more about that later. These phases may take several hours
to change from one to the other, or they may take days—in the
case of congestive heart failure—or they may take seconds or
minutes, particularly in the presence of sepsis and gram-negative
bacteria, which are prone to produce a circulatory stagnation in
selected areas of the body. The rapidity of this vasoconstrictive
reaction is endotoxin dose-related.

It is well to recall that this reaction in the microcirculation is
not a generalized one. Usually, it occurs in body areas that are
sensitive to vasoconstrictive substances or catecholamines such
as epinephrine and norepinephrine. Endotoxin itself, when it com-
bines with some constituent of the blood, is a sympathomimetic

type of substance. Anything that has a sympathomimetic effect usually causes constriction in the viscerocutaneous circulation. Certain other areas, such as the voluntary muscles, are relatively insensitive to catalytic agents as well as to most other substances, whether they be vasodilator or vasoconstrictor. This selective response, we believe, is the link in various types of shock. Indeed, it may be first aid, or nature's remedy, so to speak. Perhaps the reason there is such a high mortality in certain types of shock is damage to sensitive areas such as the kidney, lung, gut, or liver, as a result of ischemia. Moreover, a wide variety of experiments indicates that hemorrhagic, septic, and cardiogenic shock states are closely related. This relationship can be seen from microcirculatory findings, and also from tolerance-type experiments, in which, for example, dogs made tolerant to epinephrine are then found to be very tolerant to usually lethal injections of endotoxin or even to a usually fatal myocardial infarction. Endotoxin will generally produce the same result, and I think this observation further pulls the common types of shock together.

Commonly, then, in shock there is a deficiency in the effective circulating blood volume, and it may be necessary to add to the volume, or mobilize volume which is stagnant. This latter condition is, of course, characteristic of cardiogenic shock, congestive failure, and certain types of septic shock. Something has to be done to this disturbed microcirculation, and for this purpose steroids can be effective if used in the massive dosage described by Dr. Melby.

The steroids can be compared with alpha-adrenergic-blocking agents, such as phenoxybenzamine or phentolamine, or with a vasostimulator such as isoproterenol, which causes vasodilatation, primarily, it seems, in the muscular circulation. Corticosteroids are like adrenergic-blocking agents but they apparently work in different ways. Dog-paw experiments done by Dr. R. Dietzman in our laboratory seem to indicate that corticosteroids do not block receptors but they retard transmission in the sympathetic postganglionic nerve endings. In general, we see a very close relationship between these three different types of drugs. We found the corticosteroids perhaps the most useful for the clinician because they are available, they are easy to give, and can be given in a single dose.

HEMORRHAGIC SHOCK

We are now using a small portable monitoring shock unit, the type that can be pushed to the bedside of the patient. I will briefly characterize certain results that we have had in the past couple of years with this type of unit. Hemorrhagic shock is not too much of a problem. In general, it is a condition in which low volume requires volume replacement. It is the rare patient who dies in pure late, or stagnant, hemorrhagic shock. Occasionally, a vaso-dilating drug has to be given, particularly when the condition is complicated by congestive failure, but in general this is not necessary. Volume alone is usually sufficient. The readings obtained mirror exactly those that would be expected from laboratory studies of generally elevated resistance, with resistance dropping as volume is restored, elevated cardiac index with increased venous return, and, of course, a better viscerocutaneous circulation, as exemplified by warm pink skin and adequate urine output (25 or 30 cc/hr or more). The metabolic aspect is similar as volume is restored; oxygen consumption goes up; the lactic acid level may temporarily rise, due to wash-out, but then it falls to normal limits. In general, the condition can be expected to go from a constricted, ischemic type to one of a well-perfused micro-circulation, indicated by the warm pink skin and the adequate urine output. I emphasize those signs again and again because, from a clinical standpoint, I believe that an adequate urine output and good warm skin are worth all the measurements in the world.

ENDOTOXIC SHOCK

With septic shock, the problem becomes a little more compli-cated, because the clinical and the experimental situations differ; the experimental situation does not exactly mirror the clinical. In the laboratory, we generally give our dogs endotoxin from killed bacteria, whereas the patient is suffering a septicemia from living bacteria that are dying and releasing endotoxin. In general, there are two parts to the disease: one, a relatively low cardiac output, and the other, somewhat elevated or normal peripheral resistance, but the outward manifestations are the same. Generally the patient has oliguria, cold pale extremities, and is disoriented. To restore circulation, we usually give hydrocortisone in doses of 50 mg/kg of body weight—a considerably higher dosage than Dr. Melby mentioned. As a matter of fact, recent work with our patients would indicate that to get the maximum amount of vasodilatation or drop in peripheral resistance, dosage probably should be 150 mg/kg of body weight with hydrocortisone or one of the synthetics such as methylprednisolone, 30 mg/kg. With 50 mg/kg the beginning of any effect of redistribution of flow can be obtained. No remarkable effect on the cardiac index will occur, but rather a redistribution of that index, with greater urine output and gradually falling resistance. The effect usually is apparent within one to two hours. We give this dosage as a single bolus from a syringe, but it may be infused a little more slowly if desired; however, it should always be given intravenously. We have not seen any adverse effects from giving a single bolus and it has the advantage of being simple and quick.

Low Cardiac Output

We have often had patients with the low-output type of septic shock in which the resistance generally is somewhat elevated or in the high-normal range, and the cardiac index is low. Usually, central venous pressure tends to be low or normal, but volumes can be variable. We then give fluids in large volumes, basing the amount on the central venous pressure and the body weight of the patient. Our vasodilator of choice is one of the steroids. Now that the synthetics are available, our choice would be methylprednisolone in a dosage of 30 mg/kg of body weight, or dexamethasone 6 mg/kg. These are given as a single bolus. Usually, we have not repeated the dose, since the response occurs within two hours. If within four to six hours the patient does not respond, generally there are other problems, such as a perforated viscus, some hidden complication—myocardial infarction for example.

High Cardiac Output

Another type of septic shock that has attracted a good deal of interest is that associated with a high cardiac output or a high index with low peripheral resistance, yet these patients have the same peripheral manifestations of ischemia as are seen with a low cardiac output and high resistance. They are cold and clammy; they are oliguric. There may be a very early prodromal stage when they may be somewhat warmer than would be expected, but generally the outward manifestations of this type of high-output septic shock do not differ greatly from those of the low-output type.

An example of this is a patient who was hypotensive, oliguric, with cardiac output in the range of 8 to 12 liters per minute, certainly well above normal, and yet producing urine only after treatment. This patient received a total of 8 gm of hydrocortisone over a six-hour period. Blood pressure was variable. The cardiac output eventually stabilized at about 6 or 8 liters/min. Central venous pressure was raised along with volume, resistance dropping to very low levels. For that matter, it had been low initially. The apparent reason for this is shunting, which Dr. Weil has described as occurring in patients with cirrhosis. Other investigators have also found that this shunting phenomenon in the lung or the peritoneum is probably also a cause of the high cardiac output. The point is, there is still a maximal amount of constriction. As a result, the blood is going through shunts rather than through nutritive channels.

Another patient with a relatively low resistance had a cardiac arrest. He was treated with dexamethasone, I think in a dose of about 2.5 to 3.0 mg/kg of body weight. We have since found that to get maximum vasodilatation at least 6 mg/kg is required. The question may arise as to how to recognize when vasodilatation has been attained. In these patients, if, after they have been treated with one of the steroids (methylprednisolone or dexamethasone), infusion of phenoxybenzamine and a known alpha-adrenergic-blocking agent produces no further change in peripheral resistance, we then feel we have achieved a definite lowering of total peripheral resistance by means of steroids. I do not think there is any appreciable difference in the effect of the various synthetic glucocorticoids, if they are given in equivalent dosages. Small differences are seen in the laboratory, but, clinically, so far, we cannot see that one is better than another.

It is said that the mortality for the high-output type of septic shock is near, if not actually, 100%. In our own small series, however, we have had as good a response to treatment of the high-output septic shock as of the low-output type; that is, about 60% survival with steroid therapy. Based on what general experience exists, including our own, the over-all mortality with septic shock is between 60% and 80%, depending on how shock is defined.

In treating shock of any type, volume is a prime necessity. The cardiac index needs to be raised. Resistance, no matter what the figure, will generally decrease with effective treatment in the high-output type. What is essential, apparently, is a redistribution of the cardiac output. By lowering resistance and controlling infection, these arteriovenous shunts seem to close. As the patient improves, the oxygen consumption will rise, the lactic acid will wash out, and resistance will fall back to normal. So far, we have seen no prognostic value in the concentration of lactic acid. Some investigators believe that lactic acid values of 100 mg/100 cc or more, mean 100% fatality. But we have seen recovery in patients with lactic acid levels as high as 150 to 180 mg/100 cc.

CARDIOGENIC SHOCK

The third major type of shock is, of course, cardiogenic shock. Myocardial infarction in shock is one of the leading causes of death, especially in males. We have not had much experience with myocardial infarction as a cause of cardiogenic shock, and I will confine my remarks on cardiogenic shock to that which occurs primarily after open-heart surgery. We often call this low-output syndrome instead of cardiogenic shock. On the whole, it is a different type of cardiogenic shock; a damage to the pump from one cause or another—either chronic damage plus the damage of surgery, or iatrogenic valve replacement problems, with obstruction.

For example, a patient with rheumatic heart disease, mitral stenosis, and a Starr-Edwards prosthesis, goes into a low-output syndrome soon after surgery. He is cold, pale, oliguric, with high peripheral resistance, low cardiac index, and central venous pressure around 19 mm Hg. The patient is digitalized but still does not show much of a response. In the past, treatment of this type of condition with the vasopressors did not save many patients. We have now chosen to treat these patients in much the same way as I described for septic shock, that is, with massive doses of steroids, methylprednisolone 30 mg/kg body weight. After administration of the steroid there is a fall in peripheral resistance and a rise in cardiac index. The patient might also be given fluids when the central venous pressure falls, as it usually does, because we are increasing the capacity of the vascular bed. The fluids may be as important in cardiogenic shock as they are in hemorrhagic or septic shock.

As the microcirculation improves with this type of steroid therapy—this massive dose, 30 mg/kg given as a single bolus—usually oxygen consumption rises and the lactic acid level falls. Recent studies in the measurement of catecholamines in plasma and tissues have shown a general correlation between norepinephrine and epinephrine levels and the state of circulation. The higher the concentration of these catecholamines, the poorer the tissue perfusion. It has been found that after massive steroid therapy these catecholamine concentrations were decreased both in the tissues and in the plasma.

I can cite still another type of situation: Following an aortic and mitral valve replacement, the patient exhibited the low-output syndrome, with oliguria; he was pale, cold, clammy, with very high peripheral resistance (over 3,000 units), the cardiac index down about one liter, central venous pressure approaching 9 to 10 mm Hg. Here again we used a dose of methylprednisolone, 30 mg/kg body weight, and added fluids (dextran or blood or plasma). The important thing is fluid volume, and whether to use blood or not would depend on the hematocrit reading. We also use positive inotropic drugs such as isoproterenol, but we have found that this agent, used alone to resuscitate the patient in shock —either septic or cardiogenic—is not very satisfactory. After first giving steroids, however, we find that we can give a much smaller dose of isoproterenol, thus reducing the incidence of arrhythmias and other such problems that this inotropic agent can cause. The drugs in combination are more effective for the patient. Metaraminol can also be used in such a case because, while its peripheral constricting effects on the alpha-receptors are apparently blocked by the methylprednisolone—as they are by phenoxybenzamine or other alpha-adrenergic-blocking agents—its positive inotropic effect is still active. Whether we use these agents, isoproterenol or metaraminol, after steroid therapy depends to some extent on the patient's response to the steroids themselves. When there is a good response in cardiac output, we do not use an adrenergic-blocking agent.

"Washout" Effect

A rather interesting phenomenon that we see quite often, particularly in those patients in rather severely constricted circulatory states is the rise in lactic acid concentration after a vasodilator or methylprednisolone is given. Apparently, a "washout" effect occurs from the underperfused viscerocutaneous circulation, and then a fall to normal levels. The patient can be tested, in a sense, to find out what dosage of steroid produces maximum vasodilation; this, of course, is why the steroid is being used—to increase circulation. In a patient given methylprednisolone, peripheral resistance can be measured by adding a dose of phenoxybenzamine. If there is no further drop in peripheral resistance, the maximal vasodilatation has occurred. It is possible then to give epinephrine without any effect on the peripheral resistance; either epinephrine or metaraminol can be used for an inotropic effect.

To summarize our findings with cardiogenic shock, in a number of patients having the general symptoms and signs of high venous pressure, low cardiac index, and high peripheral resistance, we have observed that cardiogenic shock, like hemorrhagic shock, very closely resembles the configuration that is obtained in laboratory studies.

As circulation improves hemodynamically, oxygen consumption and the metabolic status are improved.

I mentioned that it is nice to have the clinical data indicating the patient's response, as reflected in the calculations, the indexes, the total peripheral resistance, and that sort of information; but to me, the patient's warm pink skin—in contrast to the under-perfused, pale or cyanotic skin—is, along with a good urine out-put, one of the best signs of improvement in shock, and, I believe, an underappreciated one. It takes no equipment, no technicians: simply the physician's awareness.

Survival Rate

Finally, our survival studies in various types of shock showed that for those patients who would be considered in late or stagnant shock, the mortality was in the range of 60% to 100%. We feel that with the use of vasodilators and blood volume replacement the survival rate has shown a positive increase in these three types of shock. The problem is in cardiogenic shock due to myocardial infarction, and we hope that within the year we will have a sta-tistical analysis of a study of myocardial infarction in shock in two of the large hospitals in Minneapolis and St. Paul. Conse-quently, we can get some information on the use of corticosteroids in massive dosage in the patient suffering from cardiogenic shock caused by a myocardial infarction. In extensive laboratory studies in dogs with myocardial infarction, we have had very favorable results. Moreover, in a few humans with shock due to infarction we have had similar results.

The Cardiovascular System

WILLIAM C. SHOEMAKER, M.D.

ROBERT S. BROWN, M.D.

PATRICIA A. MOHR, M.D.

DAVID O. MONSON, M.D.

JOSEPH S. CAREY, M.D.

Glucocorticoids, which have been widely used in many areas of clinical medicine, have recently been applied to the therapy of clinical shock syndromes. Sambhi, Weil and Udhoji[1] measured cardiac output and intravascular pressures in nine septic shock patients before and after administration of large doses of glucocorticoids. This agent produced sustained increases in cardiac output and decreased peripheral resistance; there were no statistically significant changes in arterial or venous pressures.

Wilson and Fisher[2] recently reported observations on the hemodynamic effects of massive doses of steroids given to 23 patients in septic shock. No over-all statistical analysis was presented, but these authors stated that steroid therapy increased cardiac output 23% in 30 minutes and 19% after one hour; thereafter, cardiac outputs fell below control values. The response was greater in patients who had initial low cardiac outputs with high peripheral

This study was supported by USPHS Grants HE 08512 and GM 15694, by USPHS Research Career Award 1K6–HE–6305 from the National Heart Institute, and by U.S. Army Contract DADA–17–69–9089.

16

resistances. Cardiac function, that is, cardiac output relative to inflowing venous pressure, did not appear to be altered by steroids.

The present preliminary studies were undertaken to explore the effect of hydrocortisone given to a random group of shock patients for whom trauma was the major etiologic event. The hemodynamic responses to hydrocortisone were compared with other agents commonly employed in shock therapy.

CLINICAL MATERIAL

The cardiovascular effects of hydrocortisone therapy were observed in a series of 16 studies in an unselected group of 12 shock patients. The clinical features of the series are summarized in Table I. The series includes three patients with uncomplicated septic shock, four patients who had sustained trauma, and five patients with a combination of hemorrhage, trauma, and sepsis as the etiologic events. The mean arterial blood pressure of the series averaged 51 mm Hg at the time of the maximum hypotension and 75 mm Hg immediately prior to hydrocortisone administration. At the time of the studies, the mean control cardiac outputs of two patients were low (less than 2.5 1/min/M^2), eight were high (greater than 4.0 1/min M^2) and six were normal or nearly normal. Eight of the patients died, six during the period of shock and two after subsequent operations. Of this group of 12 patients only four survived. Hemodynamic data before and after hydrocortisone therapy was compared with data from a series of 17 normal healthy subjects who had no evidence of cardiovascular disease.

CARDIOVASCULAR MEASUREMENTS

The methods used in these studies have been reported in detail.[3,4] Briefly, intravascular pressures were measured directly with Statham pressure transducers and recorded on an Offner multiple channel recorder. Central venous pressures were obtained from a

TABLE I. SUMMARY OF CLINICAL DATA FOR 12 SHOCK PATIENTS

Patient No.	Age	Sex	Etiology	Degree of Severity	Lowest Mean Arterial Pressure	Diagnosis	Operation	Outcome
15	48	M	Hemorrhage, trauma, sepsis	Severe	47	Gunshot wound of abdomen; perforated stomach, duodenum, jejunum, and inferior mesenteric vein	Resection of jejunal segment, closure of stomach, repair of vein	Died
40	36	F	Trauma	Moderate	53	Cirrhosis; esophageal varices with hemorrhage	Portacaval shunt	Survived
78	52	F	Trauma	Mild	75	Carcinoma of breast	Adrenalectomy	Died after subsequent operation
81	39	M	Sepsis, trauma, hemorrhage	Severe	37	Perforated duodenal ulcer	Closure of perforated peptic ulcer	Died
85	53	M	Sepsis, trauma, hemorrhage	Severe	38	Bladder carcinoma; dehiscence	Ideal diversion; closure of dehiscence	Died

Patient No.	Age	Sex	Etiology	Degree of Severity	Lowest Mean Arterial Pressure	Diagnosis	Operation	Outcome
88	28	F	Sepsis	Severe	47	Septic abortion	D & C	Survived
94	52	M	Sepsis, hemorrhage, trauma	Severe	48	Gunshot wound of abdomen; perforated bowel	Closure of perforated ileum	Died
95	45	M	Head injury	Moderate	70	Head injury; basal skull fracture	None	Survived
96	37	F	Sepsis	Severe	37	Septic abortion	None	Survived
173	18	F	Sepsis	Severe	60	Septic abortion	Hysterectomy	Died
212	75	M	Trauma	Severe	40	Multiple trauma; fractured ankle and maxilla; basal skull fracture; flail chest, pneumothorax	None	Died
222	30	F	Sepsis, trauma, hemorrhage	Moderate	60	Septic abortion; perforated uterus	Hysterectomy	Died

long plastic catheter placed in the right atrium or superior vena cava via percutaneous puncture of the brachial or subclavian veins. Plastic catheters were placed, percutaneously, in the femoral artery using six-inch No. 17 thin-wall needles for direct arterial pressure measurements and arterial blood sampling.

Cardiac output measurements were made by means of the Stewart-Hamilton Method.[5] Approximately 3.5 mg of indocyanine green were injected rapidly into the central venous catheter; arterial dye concentrations of indocyanine green were measured, calibrated and recorded with a Gilford photodensitometer and an Offner recorder. Sterilized Teflon tubing was used in all connections, so that the patient's blood could be replaced after each determination. The cardiac output and derived data from the dye curves were calculated by the formula:

$$\text{Cardiac Output} = \frac{\text{amount of dye injected}}{\int_0^\infty c(t)\, dt};$$

where t is time and $c(t)$ is the arterial concentration of the dye as a function of time. The mean transit time was calculated with the following formula:

$$\text{Mean Transit Time} = \frac{\int_0^\infty t c(t)\, dt}{\int_0^\infty c(t)\, dt}.$$

An LGP-30 digital computer programmed for this purpose was used to make these calculations. Total peripheral resistances and stroke volumes were calculated according to standard formulae.

Protocol

Prior to administration of steroid therapy, two to five control measurements were made during relatively stable periods when the patient did not exhibit anxiety, restlessness, or agitation. In nine studies, hydrocortisone sodium succinate in doses of approximately 5 mg/kg body weight were administered intravenously; in two studies 15 mg/kg were given, and in five studies approximately 50 mg/kg were given. Two to eight measurements were made at intervals up to three hours after administration of hydrocortisone. For comparative purposes all values were expressed in terms of surface area. Hydrocortisone was given late in the course of shock to only two patients.

RESULTS

The hemodynamic data from the series of shock patients before and after hydrocortisone therapy is summarized in Table II. In this table the mean values for mean arterial pressure, heart rate, central venous pressure, cardiac index, mean transit time, stroke index and peripheral resistance of the normal subjects are compared with those of the shock patients before and after hydrocortisone therapy.

Prior to hydrocortisone therapy the group of shock patients had decreased mean femoral arterial pressure, and peripheral resistance, as well as increased heart rate, central venous pressure, cardiac index, and mean transit time. The mean hemodynamic values of the shock series obtained before hydrocortisone administration were statistically not significantly different from values after hydrocortisone therapy.

The time-course of these variables is illustrated in Figure 1. No particular temporal pattern was seen after hydrocortisone administration.

When each study was examined individually, relatively small

TABLE II. HEMODYNAMIC DATA OF NORMAL SUBJECTS AND OF SHOCK PATIENTS BEFORE AND AFTER HYDROCORTISONE THERAPY

	Normal Subjects	Shock Patients	
		Before Therapy	After Therapy
Mean femoral arterial pressure (mm Hg)	92 ± 1.1	$74.2 \pm 5.1*$	71.4 ± 5.6
Heart rate (beats/min)	71 ± 1.6	102.8 ± 6.8	103.6 ± 5.9
Central venous pressure (cm H_2O)	6.1 ± 0.4	9.7 ± 2.4	10.5 ± 2.4
Cardiac index (L/min/M^2)	3.19 ± 0.05	4.64 ± 0.62	4.50 ± 0.59
Mean transit time (sec)	13.3 ± 0.3	15.6 ± 1.6	17.1 ± 2.3
Stroke index (ml/M^2)	46 ± 1.1	46.2 ± 4.8	45.2 ± 4.4
Total peripheral resistance (dyne·cm/sec^5/M^2)	2178 ± 57	1476 ± 182	1699 ± 248

* Mean and standard error of the mean.

changes were observed. There was increased cardiac output in three patients. One patient with septicemia had a high cardiac index which responded (16% increase) to the 5 mg/kg dose of hydrocortisone. The second patient, who had sustained multiple injuries, had normal output values which responded (32% increase) to the low dosage of hydrocortisone, but did not improve with the high dosage. The third patient, who sustained a head injury, had a normal cardiac output value which responded (46%) to the 50 mg/kg dose. The greatest increase was observed

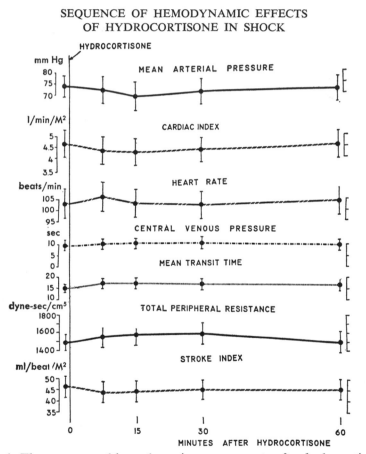

Fig 1. The sequence of hemodynamic measurements after hydrocortisone therapy is illustrated. Dots represent mean values, and cross bars the standard error of the means of the series.

TABLE III. CARDIAC INDEX RESPONSE TO HYDROCORTISONE THERAPY RELATIVE TO CONTROL VALUES

Patients with:	Mean Values	
	Before Therapy	After Therapy
Low cardiac index	1.84 1/min/M^2	1.82 1/min/M^2
Normal cardiac index	3.09 1/min/M^2	3.05 1/min/M^2
High cardiac index	6.32 1/min/M^2	6.27 1/min/M^2

TABLE IV. CARDIAC INDEX RESPONSES TO VARIOUS DOSES OF HYDROCORTISONE THERAPY

Dose	Before Therapy	After Therapy
5 mg/kg	3.66 1/min/M^2	3.54 1/min/M^2
15 mg/kg	5.96 1/min/M^2	6.2 1/min/M^2
50 mg/kg	5.69 1/min/M^2	5.53 1/min/M^2

TABLE V. CARDIAC INDEX RESPONSE TO HYDROCORTISONE RELATIVE TO ETIOLOGY OF SHOCK

	Before Therapy	After Therapy
Trauma	4.02 1/min/M^2	4.41 1/min/M^2
Sepsis	3.64 1/min/M^2	3.94 1/min/M^2
Trauma, sepsis and hemorrhage	4.02 1/min/M^2	4.41 1/min/M^2

in the patient who had the mildest hypotension. Three patients had decreased cardiac outputs after hydrocortisone therapy; these decrements were 17%, 35%, and 57% of control values.

We did not observe differences in the hemodynamic responses with respect to the dose of hydrocortisone, the etiologic type of shock, the control cardiac index value, the stage of shock or the degree of hypotension (Tables III to V). Since this is a relatively small series of patients representing a wide variety of shock syndromes, the conclusions must be considered tentative. Nevertheless, we were unable to document a statistically significant hemodynamic response.

Steroid Effect

The failure of the data of the present study to confirm significantly increased cardiac outputs in shock patients after steroid therapy is somewhat disparate from previously reported studies. There are several explanations for this apparent difference. Sambhi et al.[1] and Wilson and Fisher[2] studied predominantly septicemic patients, but only three of 16 studies of the present series were obtained in patients in whom shock was primarily attributable to sepsis. In addition, previous reports[1,2] suggested that improved cardiac output after steroid therapy occurred in those patients whose shock was characterized by low cardiac outputs and high total peripheral resistances. In the present studies only two patients had low cardiac outputs at the time of steroid therapy. The effects of steroids may not be uniform or predictable because of widely different patterns of hemodynamic changes that have been demonstrated in unselected series of shock patients.[6]

The failure to observe significant hemodynamic responses to steroid therapy in the present series may be interpreted as indicating that the patients were in a late stage of shock and unresponsive to all modes of therapy. The relative effectiveness of various types of therapy is an important question which must be answered by comparative studies on large series of patients. In clinical shock states, it is essential to have some basis of comparison for evaluating various forms of therapy. As an approach to this problem, we first made the assumption that no two shock patients are exactly alike and, second, we gave specific agents in random order so that the patient would serve as his own control.

Dextran-40 Effect

Our initial investigations were concerned with measurement of hemodynamic responses of dextran-40 in a series of 24 patients with shock of varying etiologies.[7] All patients were given 500 ml of dextran-40 intravenously; measurements were made before, during and for two to four hours after the infusion. The time course of hemodynamic response of the shock patients was compared with that of normal subjects (Fig 2). Normal subjects have a small but statistically significant increase in their cardiac index. The shock patients almost doubled their cardiac index; the transit time and central venous pressure improved. There was redistribution of blood volume, so that more of the blood returned from the peripheral small vessels into the central blood volume; the latter is the volume between the central venous catheter and the femoral arterial catheter.

In addition we[8] have compared cardiorespiratory responses in a series of 11 patients in traumatic shock who were given equal volumes (500 ml) of dextran-40 and whole blood in random order (Fig 3 and 4). Various hemodynamic and pulmonary functional measurements were taken in a control period and continued during and after volume loading. Dextran significantly increased cardiac output and oxygen consumption in traumatic and hemor-

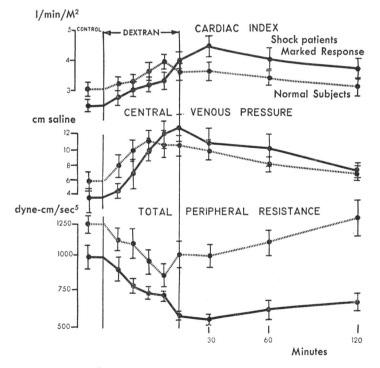

Fig 2. Hemodynamic responses to Dextran-40 in a series of 6 normal subjects and 24 patients in shock from a combination of hemorrhage, trauma, and sepsis. The time-course of changes in cardiac index, central venous pressure and peripheral resistance before, during, and after infusion of 500 ml of Dextran-40 is shown. Dots represent mean values, and bars the standard error of the mean. Data from Mohr et al.[7]

rhagic shock; blood increased only output. We observed that neither blood nor dextran improved oxygen consumption in a small group of patients with septicemia or septic shock.

Further, the response to randomly administered plasma expanders was compared in patients who were in normovolemic shock; that is, they may have had blood loss at one time, but their blood volumes had been restored to the normal range at the time of the study. Responses to dextran-40, dextran-70, albumin,

EFFECT OF DEXTRAN-40 IN TRAUMATIC SHOCK

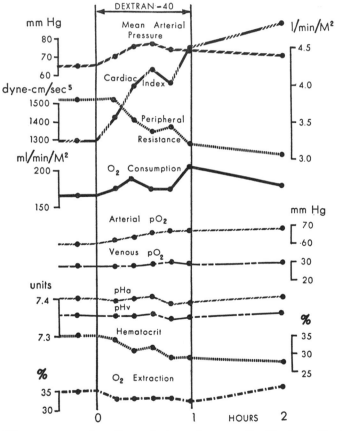

Fig 3. The sequence of cardiorespiratory changes after Dextran-40 administration in a series of patients with traumatic shock are shown. The average values of the series are shown before, during, and after 500 ml of Dextran-40 was administered. Data from Kho and Shoemaker.[8]

plasma, whole blood and saline were compared (Fig 5). From the standpoint of cardiac output, the plasma expanders generally gave a much greater hemodynamic response than did whole blood.[9]

Vasopressors

The vasopressors also have been studied by many investigators, with the result that there are conflicting reports on their usefulness

EFFECT OF BLOOD IN TRAUMATIC SHOCK

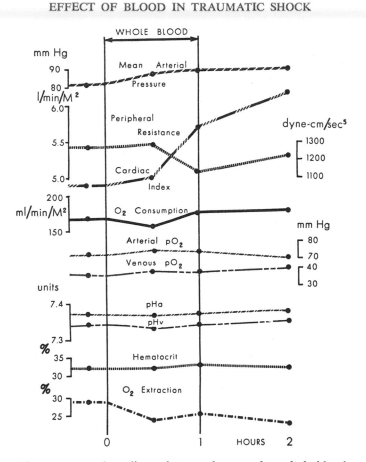

Fig 4. The sequence of cardiorespiratory changes after whole blood transfusion in the traumatic shock group are shown. The average values of the series are shown before, during, and after a 500-ml blood transfusion.

CARDIAC OUTPUT RESPONSES TO BLOOD
AND PLASMA VOLUME EXPANDERS

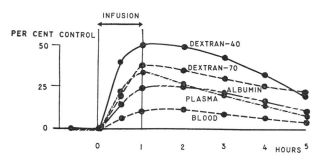

Fig 5. Time sequence of cardiac output responses to 500 ml of Dextran-40, Dextran-70, albumin, plasma, and whole blood given over a one-hour period in random order to a series of patients whose blood volumes were normal or near normal. Data from Carey et al.[9]

and their appropriateness. We[10] have attempted to resolve this problem by studying the hemodynamic responses to representative sympathomimetic agents in a systematic manner. Figure 6 illustrates the comparative changes in 17 patients, most of whom had a combination of septic, traumatic, and hemorrhagic shock. The patients were given norepinephrine, metaraminol, methoxamine, and isoproterenol in random order. It may be seen that, in the patient whose shock arises from multiple etiologies, there are greater increases in cardiac output after isoproterenol administration than after the other agents. Furthermore, there are greater increases in cardiac output relative to the increase in cardiac work.

One definite conclusion we have drawn is that the hemodynamic alterations of shock patients differ with respect to the etiologic types of shock, the stage of shock, and the degree of shock.[6] Apparently contradictory conclusions in previously reported studies may result from comparison of data from patients with shock of various degrees, etiologies and stages. An example of this may be cited. In normovolemic shock patients, dextran-40 and other plasma expanders notably increased cardiac output, but whole blood produced minimal improvement in cardiac output. By contrast, hypovolemic patients with uncomplicated blood loss unassociated with operative trauma or sepsis respond equally well,

INCREMENTAL CHANGES IN HEMODYNAMICS AFTER SYMPATHOMIMETIC AMINES AND HYDROCORTISONE

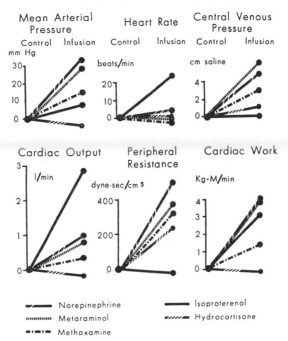

Fig 6. Changes in arterial pressure, heart rate, central venous pressure, cardiac output, peripheral resistance, and cardiac work in a series of 17 shock patients given constant infusions of norepinephrine, metaraminol, methoxamine, and isoproterenol in random order; data from Brown et al.[10] Comparison is made with the response to hydrocortisone of the present study.

in hemodynamic terms, to whole blood transfusions or dextran-40 infusions.[3]

Sequential Pattern

It is of utmost importance to appreciate the natural history of hemodynamic alterations which progressively develop over the time-course of shock arising from various etiologic types. On the basis of more than 10,000 hemodynamic measurements in 240 critically ill patients, we have characterized the various sequential patterns of hemodynamic events in shock occurring from various etiologies (Fig 7). Moreover, we have identified certain factors that increase or decrease cardiac output. Some anesthetic agents, such as cyclopropane, tend to increase cardiac output in shock patients, but barbiturates tend to decrease it. Obviously, dehydration and hypovolemia diminish cardiac output; they are probably a major cause of reduced output early in the course of hemorrhagic and septic shock. In traumatic, burn, and uncomplicated septic shock, there are usually increased outputs through most of their course. In the terminal stages—that is, immediately prior to death—most patients had low outputs.

The majority of patients we see in the common clinical setting can not be classified into these pure etiologic categories, but have shock associated with multiple causes. They are usually the patients who have been subjected to blood loss from operations and then have postoperative complications, such as sepsis and pulmonary problems. This group with mixed etiologies predomi-

CARDIAC INDEX PATTERNS IN VARIOUS TYPES OF SHOCK

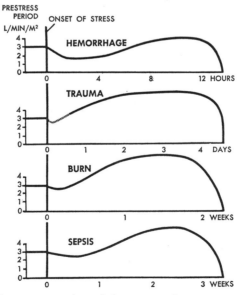

Fig 7. Schematic representation of the temporal sequence of cardiac index changes in shock induced by uncomplicated hemorrhage, trauma, burns and sepsis.

nantly have patterns of high cardiac output with a low peripheral resistance.

Vasodilators

Since most of the patients with shock from multiple causes have a high output with low resistance, we find it is unusual for a blocking agent to be indicated. We have used phenoxybenzamine and phentolamine. They may improve peripheral flow, as reflected by increased skin temperature and urine output. But the cerebral and the coronary vessels, which are not under sympathetic nervous system control are not directly affected by blocking agents. Therefore, when the patient is blocked, there may be relative improvement in flow to all areas except the brain and the heart. The patient may have improvement of total blood flow, only to end up with myocardiac infarction or neurological deficit. One must be aware of this problem when using blocking agents.

Over and above the statistical evaluation of the series of patients there is some merit in looking at responses of individual cases. Figure 8 illustrates the cardiac output responses in sepsis, in which two patients had septic abortions and one patient had pyelonephritis. Cardiac output values of the first patient, a 28-year-old woman with septic abortion, are illustrated by the upper section of Figure 8. There was a short-lived response to isoproterenol; then tachyphylaxis occurred. Norepinephrine and epinephrine were given without effect. Volume-loading with dextran-40 produced marked improvement in cardiac output which persisted for about two hours. Other plasma expanders, including whole blood, were given, and the patient made a satisfactory recovery. Cardiac output values of the second patient, a 37-year-old woman with septic abortion, are illustrated by the center section of Figure 8; she was given three sympathomimetic agents with modest but transient improvement. Hydrocortisone produced no significant hemodynamic change. This patient also did not respond to dextran-40. However, after volume-loading with the dextran, the response to isoproterenol was much more pronounced and more lasting. With constant infusion of this agent, the patient made a relatively uneventful recovery. Data on the third patient, a 47-year-old man with uncomplicated septic shock (pyelonephritis)—that is, without evidence of blood loss or trauma—are illustrated by the lower section of Figure 8. The initial response to isoproterenol was rela-

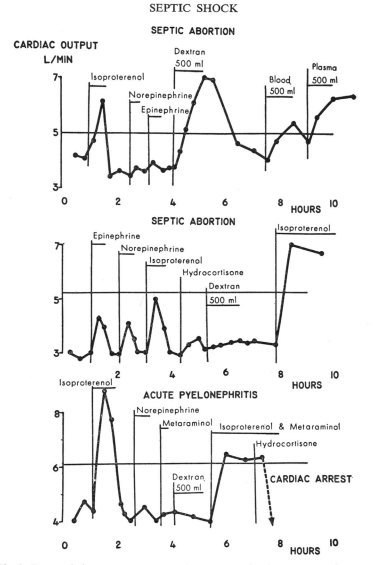

Fig 8. Data of the responses to various agents in three cases of uncomplicated septic shock.

tively short-lived and there was no response to norepinephrine, metaraminol, dextran, or a combination of isoproterenol and norepinephrine. The patient was given hydrocortisone and, following this, had a cardiac arrest.

SUMMARY

The hemodynamic response to steroid therapy was measured in 16 studies on 12 shock patients. No significant hemodynamic changes were observed in this series. In a similar population of shock patients other agents were shown to produce significant hemodynamic changes. More quantitative information is necessary to define more precisely the indications for this agent and to predict its effect. Until such information is available it would seem more appropriate in the clinical setting to use as primary therapy those agents which more consistently effect hemodynamic improvement. The lack of hemodynamic effects after hydrocortisone does not imply that there are not other beneficial effects arising from its metabolic actions.

REFERENCES

1. Sambhi, M. P., Weil, M. H., and Udhoji, V. N.: Acute Pharmacodynamic Effects of Glucocorticoids, *Circulation* **31**:523, 1965.

2. Wilson, R. F., and Fisher, R. R.: Hemodynamic Effects of Massive Steroids in Clinical Shock, *Surg. Gynec. Obstet.* **127**:769, 1968.

3. Monson, D. O., and Shoemaker, W. C.: Sequence of Hemodynamic Events After Various Types of Hemorrhage, *Surgery* **63**:738, 1968.

4. Shoemaker, W. C., Printen, K. J., Amato, J. J., Monson, D. O., Carey, J. S., and O'Connor, K.: Hemodynamic Patterns After Acute Anesthetized and Unanesthetized Trauma, *Arch. Surg.* **95**:492, 1967.

5. Hamilton, W. F., Moore, J. W., Kinsman, J. M., and Spurling, R. G.: Studies on the Circulation, *Amer. J. Physiol.* **99**:534, 1932.

6. Shoemaker, W. C., Elwyn, D. H., and Rosen, A. L.: Development and Goals of Trauma and Shock Research Center, *J. Mount Sinai Hosp.* **35**:451, 1968.

7. Mohr, P. A., Monson, D. O., Owczarski, C., and Shoemaker, W. C.: Sequential Cardiorespiratory Events During and After Dextran-40 Infusion in Normal and Shock Patients. *Circulation* **39**:379–393, 1969.

8. Kho, L. K., and Shoemaker, W. C.: Evaluation of Therapy in Clinical

Shock by Cardiorespiratory Measurements, *Surg. Gynec. Obstet.* **127**:81, 1968.

9. Carey, J. S., Brown, R. S., Woodward, N., Yao, S. T., and Shoemaker, W. C.: Comparison of Hemodynamic Responses to Whole Blood and Plasma Expanders in Clinical Traumatic Shock, *Surg. Gynec. Obstet.* **121**:563, 1965.

10. Brown, R. S., Carey, J. S., Mohr, P. A., Monson, D. O., and Shoemaker, W. C.: Comparative Evaluation of Sympathomimetic Amines in Clinical Shock, *Circulation* **34**:260, 1966.

The Vascular Smooth Muscle

JACOB FINE, M.D.

My first experience with steroid was with desoxycorticosterone in 1936. It did something startling: rabbits given trypan blue were decidedly less blue when given the corticosteroid. It altered membrane permeability. But there was not much of this steroid available then and we went no further with it.

During the last ten years or so Spink, Weil, and their colleagues have published numerous papers urging the use of corticosteroids, especially in septic shock. Most clinicians now agree that once in a while these steroids perform what appears to be a miracle; the good response is so closely linked in time to their administration that their role in the result cannot be denied. Skeptics have questioned the validity of this therapy because the proponents of corticosteroids have steadily increased the recommended dose. Perhaps the large doses can be dangerous, but something that cannot be shown to have inflicted damage and might save a life cannot be faulted, considering the stakes involved and the fact—at least from my own observations—that when steroids work at all in shock one or two large doses will suffice to reverse the deteriorating course.

Dexamethasone Effect

When we began experimenting with the steroids, we started
with dexamethasone in a dosage of 2 to 8 mg/kg of body weight,
a range used in an experimental study by Dr. Lillehei.[1] We looked
for the effect of the steroid by focusing on the hemodynamics,
rather than on lysosomes or other phenomena at the level of
molecular biology, for the latter studies are at too fundamental
a level to be useful for a clinical understanding of the cause of
death. Since the death is clearly the result of defective blood flow,
we preferred to explain the favorable hemodynamic response as
repair of a structural defect that might account for the functional
collapse of the peripheral vessels. We therefore made studies of
vascular muscle by electron microscopy.

ELECTRON-MICROSCOPIC STUDIES

Smooth muscle from a vein closely resembles arterial muscle
in electron-microscopic photographs; and for all practical purposes samples can be taken from any part of the peripheral circulation. Figure 1 shows part of a muscle cell from a vein in a state
of partial relaxation. The myofibrils are cut in longitudinal sections, and show an ordered parallel arrangement. Figure 2 shows
a section cut obliquely or transversely, so that one can see closely
packed bundles at various angles. There are dense areas in the
matrix, the nature of which is obscure, though they are said to be
analogous to the intercalated discs in striated muscle. The muscle
is contracted, as one can readily deduce from the wrinkling of
the walls of the nucleus. In Figure 3 the cell is from an animal
in advanced hemorrhagic shock. The normal pattern of the
myofibrils is lost. They are spread apart and distorted apparently
by some change in the matrix, as if water had entered or viscosity
had decreased by depolymerization of macromolecules. Figure 4
shows the plasma membrane damaged so that it allows protrusions
of cytoplasm to occur. Such muscle is not likely to function effec-
tively. Its condition fits the hemodynamic status at the time of

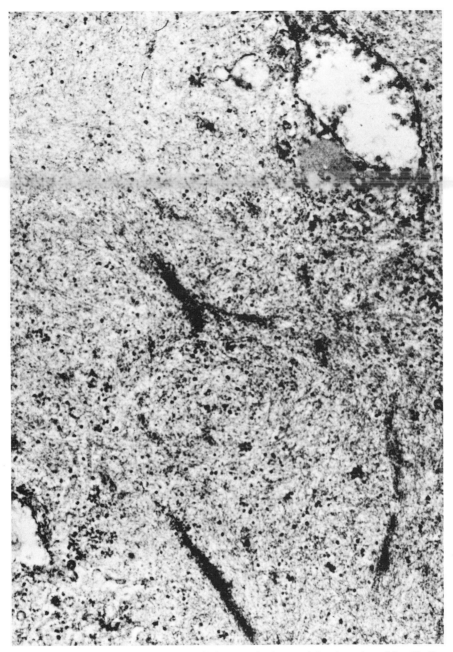

Fig 1. Section of animal muscle cell from vein in partial relaxation. Myofibrils, cut in longitudinal section, reveal ordered parallel arrangement. ($\times$33,750)

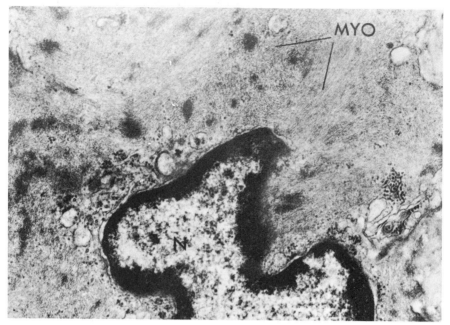

Fig 2. Section of animal muscle from vein cut obliquely, visualizing closely packed bundles at various angles, and dense areas in matrix. Wrinkled walls of nucleus indicate contracted muscle. (×33,750)

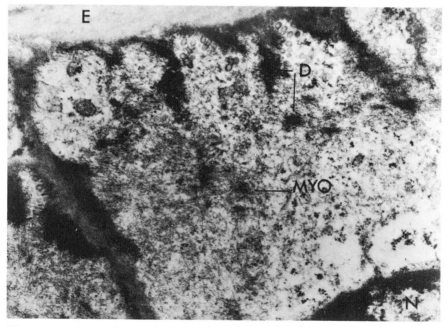

Fig 3. Muscle cell from animal in advanced hemorrhagic shock. Myofibrils distorted and spread apart, suggesting water had entered, or depolymerization of macromolecules had decreased viscosity. (×27,000)

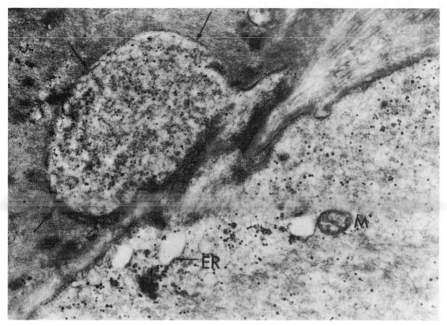

Fig. 4. Damaged plasma membrane with protrusions of cytoplasm. ($\times$27,000)

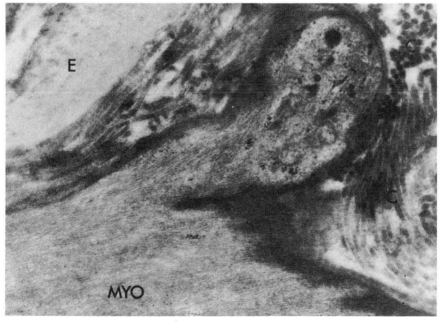

Fig 5. Vascular muscle from animal responding favorably to steroid therapy. Cytoplasm restored; myofibrils arranged normally. Cytoplasm normal in still unretracted protrusions through plasma membrane. ($\times$27,000)

TABLE I. EFFECT OF DEXAMETHASONE ON HEMODYNAMICS OF ENDOTOXIC SHOCK IN DOGS

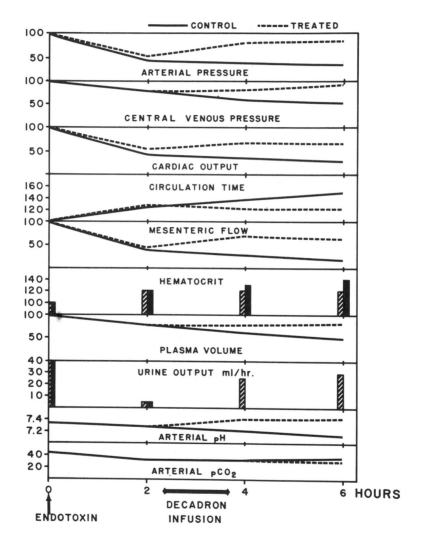

sampling, when mesenteric flow is less than a third of normal and the cardiac output is falling steadily (Table I).

Formerly we would have regarded this as an irreversible situation, and expected the animal to die within a few hours. At this critical point, no amount of blood or other conventional therapy will work, but a buffered saline solution containing a huge dose of dexamethasone (8 mg/kg), infused over a period of an hour or two, effects a change in the right direction, so that after some time the animal shows progressive improvement. Figure 5 shows the vascular muscle one or two hours after favorable response to steroid. The cytoplasm is restored to normal, and the myofibrils are arranged normally. Even in the protrusion through the plasma membrane, which has not yet retracted, the cytoplasm is back to normal. Since functional and structural recovery are simultaneous, the steroid can be credited with the hemodynamic recovery. No other therapy is needed to restore normal flow. Even if there is a substantial plasma or whole blood volume deficit, improvement will be progressive and transfusion will not be required.

LIMITATIONS OF STEROID THERAPY

The limitations of steroid therapy must be understood in order to properly assess what can be expected of it. Thus, immediate recovery from shock after steroid therapy is no assurance of sustained survival; in our experimental animal studies most 24-hour survivors died within the next 5 to 7 days. This demonstrates that mere prolongation of survival time for hours or for a few days is not enough. Only a therapy which achieves sustained recovery is of telling significance. The fact that a sufficiently large dose of dexamethasone, followed by four days of antibiotic therapy, achieves such a cure, though neither drug alone can do this, signifies that steroid can correct the hemodynamic disorder but cannot restore the antibacterial defense; and that complete recovery requires that the latter be protected by antibiotic therapy against further injury during the recovery period.

The response to steroid also hinges on the degree of resistance to shock. This varies with the history of prior exposure to trauma and infection and the degree and duration of shock prior to administering the steroid. One can see the degree of resistance to shock in animals when they are exposed to hemorrhagic shock by the elevated reservoir technic. The rate at which blood in the reservoir is reclaimed is a measure of resistance. The nonresistant animal begins to reclaim blood within some 30 minutes because of failing compensatory vasoconstriction, and frequently will, within several hours, have reclaimed over half of the total lost, after which transfusion of the remainder produces only a transient pressor response. If such an animal is treated with steroid and recovers, and is exposed again within the next few weeks to the same degree of hemorrhagic shock, it will reclaim very little, or at least much less, blood from the reservoir and will not need steroids to recover hemodynamic balance. The ability to sustain vascular tone is better than during the first exposure, and is a measure of increased resistance.

The same increase in resistance can be induced by a series of injections of endotoxin. This increase in resistance to shock as well as to endotoxin is lost after some 30 days. The parallels between resistance to shock and to endotoxin, in degree as well as in duration, implies their interchangeability. This suggests that the integrity of vascular muscle and the antiendotoxic function of the reticuloendothelial system are interdependent.

The dose of steroid required to restore hemodynamic balance varies with the degree of resistance. Thus Table II shows a series of rabbits which took blood back rapidly and Table III shows a series that took blood back slowly. The former need a much larger dose of steroid, and require antibiotic therapy for full recovery. Those that take blood back slowly may require steroid but not antibiotic, or vice versa.

REFERENCE

1. Lillehei, R. C., and MacLean, L. D.: Physiological Approach to Successful Treatment of Endotoxin Shock in the Experimental Animal, *Arch. Surg.* **78**:464, 1959.

TABLE II. STEROID THERAPY OF HEMORRHAGIC SHOCK IN RABBITS
WITH RAPID UPTAKE*

Therapy	Number of Experiments	Survivals (%)			
		24 hr	48 hr	72 hr	168 hr
None	20	0	0	0	0
Dexamethasone, I.V. (2 mg/kg body wt)	8	37	12	0	0
Dexamethasone, I.V. (2 mg/kg body wt) plus antibiotic	8	50	38	25	12
Antibiotic	8	0	0	0	0
Dexamethasone, I.V. (4 mg/kg body wt) plus antibiotic	5	40	20	20	20
Dexamethasone, I.V. (8 mg/kg body wt)	8	25	12	12	12
Dexamethasone, I.V. (8 mg/kg body wt) plus antibiotic	16	81	81	81	81
Dexamethasone, intra-aortic (4 mg/kg body wt) plus antibiotic	21	85	81	81	81

* Therapy was started after all shed blood had returned.

TABLE III. STEROID THERAPY OF HEMORRHAGIC SHOCK IN RABBITS
WITH SLOW UPTAKE*

Therapy	Number of Experiments	Survivals (%)			
		24 hr	48 hr	72 hr	168 hr
None	5	100	0	0	0
Dexamethasone, I.V. (2 mg/kg body wt)	10	80	80	80	80
Dexamethasone, I.V. (2 mg/kg body wt) plus antibiotic	10	100	100	100	100
Antibiotic	15	93	80	74	67

* Therapy was started after all shed blood had returned.

Water and Salt Metabolism

WILLIAM DRUCKER, M.D.

This topic is a most difficult one because it is diffused. It is well known that when shock occurs, a series of homeostatic adjustments takes place. One adjustment that has been studied as intensely as any is the renal response. The phenomena of the pressor receptors in the kidney, the release of angiotensin, and the eventual activity of aldosterone with retention of salt and water as a protective device when the body fluid volume is depleted have all been studied. I should like to discuss the exchange of fluid across the capillary networks, without being too precise as to which network is being considered, recognizing quite clearly that capillaries do differ and therefore the concepts of function do not always apply uniformly.

PHYSIOLOGY OF FLUID EXCHANGE

In a discussion of the role of steroids in the capillary system, a rather logical series of questions would be: First, what is the physiology of capillary fluid exchange as we know it today? Investigation is very active in this field, and I can touch on it only in the

44

most cursory manner. The next question would be: What happens to capillary exchange during shock? And then a third question, it seems to me, would be: What happens to capillary exchange when there is adrenal insufficiency? And finally, a synthesis of the data, to try to learn what happens to the capillary exchange in an adrenal-deficient patient or animal in shock.

Most of the circulating blood volume is on the venous side and very little is actually in the capillary system. And yet, this is where the exchange occurs which either protects or fails to protect the circulating fluid volume insofar as contribution from the interstitial fluid is concerned.

There is a decline in effective capillary hydrostatic pressure in the progress from the arterial end to the venous end of a capillary. Filtration on the arterial side is into the interstitial space, because the hydrostatic pressure is greater than the effective capillary osmostic pressure which acts to retain the fluid in the capillary. At the venous end, the capillary hydrostatic pressure falls low enough for the fluid to enter the capillary circulation from the interstitium. It is in this capillary system, discussed by Dr. Lillehei, that capacitance and resistance vessels have their function. The relationship between the arterial and venous constrictions in these vessels determines to a great extent the pressure in the total capillary system. Constriction in the resistance vessels on the arterial end of the capillary reduces the head of hydrostatic pressure that would ordinarily push fluid out of the capillary. Thus less fluid is lost from the capillary, and vascular refilling is enhanced. This homeostatic response is initiated early in shock.

Contribution of Volume from Cells

In these considerations, I wish to emphasize at the outset that there is in the shock literature gross misinformation that cells contribute to the protection of fluid volume during shock. There is absolutely no evidence of this except under circumstances which promote cellular destruction, or when the osmotic pressure of the extracellular fluid increases, or under the special circumstances of adrenal insufficiency which I shall discuss shortly. It should be clear that in acute hemorrhagic shock, cells do not contribute fluid to protect circulating blood volume! The forces that allow transport of fluid across the cell membrane are osmotic forces; a change in hydrostatic pressure, as far as I know, affects only the fluid exchange between the plasma and the interstitial fluid volume.

Shock Model

In discussing shock, it would be well to define the terms. I am illustrating a model procedure which we have used for years to study hemorrhagic shock. It was derived from the model developed by Wiggers[1] at Western Reserve University. This model has of course been revised and improved by Dr. Fine[2] and others,[3] but it is essentially the same model. An animal is bled to any arbitrary pressure and kept there for a period of time. In order to keep a given pressure constant, it is necessary during the initial phase to remove periodically small amounts of blood. A study of the blood volume removed at various time intervals indicated it was necessary to remove an ever-increasing total volume of blood during the early shock period.

Dr. Fine spoke of an eventual uptake of blood from the animal; that is, in order to maintain a constant arterial pressure, it in time becomes necessary to return some of the withdrawn blood. In this shock model, after a certain amount of "uptake" or re-infusion of blood has occurred, the animal is rapidly transfused with all blood remaining in the reservoir and observation of the animal is continued. Now, the interval between the time when blood has been taken from the animal and the time when blood must be returned in order to keep arterial pressure constant, is quite variable. This is the period of tolerance to which Dr. Fine referred in discussing the problem of antecedent steroid therapy. I believe this is one of the most promising time-periods for investigation of the dynamic sequence of events that constitute the syndrome of shock. What is it that contributes to tolerance and that allows an animal to remain hypovolemic longer and longer before it is necessary to reinfuse his withdrawn blood? The amount of blood lost at any given time is an indication of the net effect of all the compensatory reactions in shock. One of these reactions is capillary refill. This is the homeostatic response that I will discuss now.

Studies of Fluid Transport

Data from Mellander and Lewis,[4] a long and sadly neglected, beautiful piece of experimental work conducted many years ago in Stockholm, Sweden, illustrate the earlier fatigue, as it were, of the resistance vessels versus the capacitance vessels. This change is what Dr. Lillehei referred to regarding steroid therapy. In an animal in shock, the capacitance vessels maintain their vasoconstrictive response much longer than do the resistance vessels. Therefore, an imbalance develops, allowing an increased hydrostatic pressure to enter the capillary network with the result of decreasing capillary refill from the interstitial volume. This change helps to explain the mechanism of loss of tolerance to hypovolemic shock—the capillaries in effect begin to "leak" fluid into the interstitial space, and peripheral resistance declines. In the shock model, the period of decompensation or "take-up" has begun and is reflected by the need to return some of the withdrawn blood to prevent a decline in arterial pressure.

Early in shock there is an increased net transport of fluid into the capillaries; later, less and less fluid enters the capillaries, and finally, a net loss of fluid occurs from the capillaries into the interstitium. This does not necessarily mean a change in capillary permeability. It is merely a difference between the hydrostatic forces and the osmotic forces. This concept has now been worked out mathematically by Rankin[5] of Duke University. Much of the confusion in the field of shock arises, I believe, because of failure to recognize that shock is a dynamic sequence of events, and by this I refer to time. One must be very clear, as Dr. Fine was, to state when the therapy is given, because therapy at one time can have an effect quite different from identical therapy given at another time. Time is a critical factor when we are talking about therapy, physiologic, or metabolic changes.

What happens with adrenal insufficiency? A practicing orthopedic surgeon in an area remote from any university came up with an idea, went to the University of Toronto, finally persuaded the professors to give him the assistance of a young medical student, and within nine months discovered insulin.[6] I refer, of course, to Sir Frederick Banting, and that story is well known.

Water Metabolism After Adrenalectomy

Until I began to read in greater depth, however, I did not know that after he had discovered insulin, Sir Frederick Banting[7] made another magnificent contribution to our medical knowledge—simultaneously with and quite independently of Rogoff and Stewart.[8] It was Banting's work that led to our early understanding of the pathophysiology of adrenal insufficiency. He showed that the more chronic changes are due to a loss of fluid from the vascular system—somewhere within other fluid compartments. I will not go into detail of what has been worked out since then, but studies by Gaudino and Levitt[9] showed that the fluid is lost into the cell during adrenal insufficiency. If an adrenalectomized animal is maintained for a period on desoxycorticosterone acetate (which was the only adrenal cortical steroid available until after World War II), followed by gradual withdrawal of treatment, studies of the partition of fluid will show that the fluid moves progressively into the cell.

In addition to this shift of fluid from the extracellular to intracellular space in adrenal insufficiency, there is a net loss of total body salt and water. Much of the argument on this question of capillary exchange in shock is due to a failure to distinguish clearly between the changes in acute adrenal insufficiency and those that occur with chronic adrenal insufficiency.

In the laboratory, what happens when the adrenal is removed and the animal is subjected to trauma or shock? A study by Marks[10] in Boston a few years ago, in which a left adrenalectomy was followed some time later by a right adrenalectomy, relates to the work started long ago by Swingle,[11] who has been working in this field for many years. Marks showed, simply, that the plasma volume declined very slightly after the left adrenalectomy. When the right adrenal was subsequently removed, the animal being then completely devoid of adrenal tissue, the plasma volume declined abruptly, at which point adrenal cortical replacement therapy was given. After this therapy, the plasma volume was restored. This restoration occurred without the administration of exogenous fluids.

Clearly, in this study the restoration of plasma volume was by an endogenous shift of fluid into the circulating blood. The blood pressure did not change during the first adrenalectomy. With the same surgeon and same operative procedure, the blood pressure declined rapidly after the second adrenalectomy, until the animal was treated with steroids. This suggests that the animal was unable to protect his plasma volume from the loss due to the trauma of surgery until adrenal steroids were replaced, and then protection for circulating volume, as indicated by blood pressure, came via the mobilization of fluid from extravascular sources. In another very clear study by Marks[10] of the changes that occur in an animal following adrenalectomy without replacement therapy, the blood pressure fell after a very mild degree of trauma, and the hematocrit rose. This indicated loss of plasma volume. It was not loss of whole blood, since the trauma was a mild degree of rubbing of the intestine. The loss of fluids or plasma from the blood resulted in a rise in hematocrit and decline in plasma volume. Steroid therapy restored a more nearly normal hematocrit; thus it promoted a shift of fluid from extravascular compartments into the bloodstream.

During hemorrhage in an adrenalectomized dog maintained on steroids, there is a fall in hematocrit due to refill of plasma volume from the capillary. Some capillary refill also results from the lymphatic flow, as demonstrated so clearly by Cope.[12] But I have no information regarding the effect of adrenal insufficiency on that homeostatic mechanism.

The same animal, subjected to shock without adrenal cortical hormone replacement therapy, undergoes a continuing depletion of plasma volume. Coupled with the fall in plasma volume is a progressive rise in hematocrit. Then, with the administration of hydrocortisone, the plasma volume comes back up even though the animal has not been given any exogenous fluids. This indicates that steroids are necessary to allow interstitial fluid to protect the plasma volume during shock.

THEORY OF EFFECT OF SHOCK

Misunderstandings may have occurred regarding the contribution of cellular fluid to protect plasma volume. My concept, subject to change with new data, is this: Adrenal insufficiency leads to a disproportionate distribution of body water, disproportionate in the sense that a greater volume of it is held within the cells. Why the fluid enters the cell I cannot say; perhaps later we can hear from Dr. Spink on this matter. Under these circumstances, with a depleted interstitial fluid volume, because it is now trapped within the cell, when an animal or human is subjected to the stress of hypovolemic shock, there is less interstitial fluid volume to help support the plasma by capillary exchange. When adrenal hormones are given, the water leaves the cells and returns to the interstitial fluid volume and then is made available via the usual forces (Starling's law) to replenish the circulating plasma volume. There are data to suggest that, additionally, these steroids, under this circumstance, have an effect on the sphincters in the capillaries, and we have just seen that in increased doses, the steroids also affect the muscles themselves. It would seem unlikely that the effect of steroid therapy on capillary refill is secondary to an action on capillary sphincters, since the mobilization of fluid occurs with steroid therapy early in shock, before the period of decompensation or presumed sphincter fatigue has developed.

I have not answered certain questions, because I do not have the answers. I do not know how the steroids act within the cell, but this is a very promising field for investigation. I do not know how the steroids act on lymph return, but lymph return is essential to plasma refill. I do not know how the steroids act on the mobilization of proteins, which must occur if plasma refill is to be effective. Otherwise, there would be plasma refill with essentially extracellular fluid without the protein. Obviously protein is necessary to preserve the osmotic forces in the capillary. Perhaps I have asked more questions than I have answered, but I do hope that I have conveyed the concept that in the presence of adrenal insufficiency in accord with mechanisms which I have discussed, a human or animal is less able to tolerate hypovolemic shock.

REFERENCES

1. Wiggers, C. J.: *Physiology of Shock* (New York: Commonwealth Fund, 1950), p. 459.

2. Fine, J., Frank, H., Schweinburg, F., Jacob, S., and Gordon, T.: The Bacterial Factor in Traumatic Shock, *Ann. New York Acad. Sc.* (art. 3) **55**:429–437, 1952.

3. Lamson, P. D., and DeTurk, W. E.: A Method for the Accurate Control of Blood Pressure, *J. Pharmacol. Exper. Ther.* **83**:250, 1945.

4. Mellander, S., and Lewis, D. H.: Effect of Hemorrhagic Shock on the Reactivity of Resistance and Capacitance Vessels and on Capillary Filtration Transfer in Cat Skeletal Muscle, *Circulation Res.* Vol. 13, 1963.

5. Rankin, E. M.: Blood Flow and Transcapillary Exchange in Skeletal Muscle, *Fed. Proc.* (no. 5, pt. 1) **24**:1092–1094, 1965.

6. De Kruif, P.: Conquest of Sugar Death; Story of Banting's Discovery of Insulin, *Ladies' Home J.* **49**:12, 1932.

7. Banting, F. G., and Gairns, S.: Suprarenal Insufficiency, *Amer. J. Physiol.* **77**:100, 1926.

8. Rogoff, J. M., and Stewart, G. N.: Studies on Adrenal Insufficiency, *Amer. J. Physiol.* **84**:649, 660, 1928.

9. Gaudino, M., and Levitt, M. F.: Influence of the Adrenal Cortex on Body Water Distribution and Renal Function, *J. Clin. Invest.* **28**:1487, 1949.

10. Marks, L. J., King, D. W., Kingsbury, P. F., Boyett, J. E., and Dell, E. S.: Physiologic Role of the Adrenal Cortex in the Maintenance of Plasma Volume Following Hemorrhage or Surgical Operation, *Surgery* **58**: 510, 1965.

11. Swingle, W. W., DaVango, J. P., Crossfield, H. C., Glenister, D., Osborne, M., Rowan, R., and Wagle, G.: Glucocorticoids and Maintenance of Blood Pressure and Plasma Volume of Adrenalectomized Dogs Subjected to Stress, *Proc. Soc. Exper. Biol. Med.* **100**:617, 1959.

12. Cope, O., and Moore, F. D.: A Study of Capillary Permeability in Experimental Burns and Burn Shock Using Radioactive Dyes in Blood and Lymph, *J. Clin. Invest.* **23**:241–257, 1944.

The Cell

WILLIAM SCHUMER, M.D.

The efficacy of corticosteroids in relieving rheumatoid symptoms, described by Hench and his colleagues[1] in 1949, led to an upsurge in corticosteroid research, but it is both chastening and disappointing that after 20 years of intensive study the mechanism of this efficacious effect is still unknown.

In 1957 Melby and co-workers[2] described the use of aldosterone in septic shock. Later, Lillehei and associates,[3] Sullivan and Cavanagh,[4] and Weil[5] urged the use of corticosteroids in cardiogenic and septic shock. Fine et al.[6] described the protective effect of steroids on the vascular muscle cells. In our laboratories we have used corticosteroids in refractory hemorrhagic shock with excellent results and are now investigating the mechanism of these effects. Since shock is a peripheral, cellular, deteriorative condition affecting the enzyme systems, we studied the microcirculatory and metabolic effects on the cells and the subsequent action of corticoids on these derangements.

In low-flow states the peripheral cells, namely the gastrointesti-

This study was supported by USPHS Research Grant No. 15614–02 from the National Institutes of Health.

nal, muscle, and skin, gradually become anoxic by progressive shunting of blood and peripheral vascular constriction. This anoxia, or histanoxia, has a profound effect on the metabolic pathways of these cells. Therefore, it seems appropriate to begin this discussion with a review of the normal cell physiology and the metabolic changes in the cell in shock.[7, 8]

METABOLIC STUDIES

The cell manufactures energy through the breakdown of glucose for the maintenance of life-sustaining chemical reactions. Glucose metabolism can produce energy along several pathways. A portion of glucose can be converted to glycogen in the liver and muscles. Glycogen is the molecule the body uses to store sugar. It is composed of an arborization of glucose units. The arborization can be debranched by the enzyme systems which are stimulated by epinephrine and glucagon to release glucose molecules for energy production.

Without oxygen, glucose can be catabolized only to pyruvate and lactic acid. When oxygen is present, further degradation of sugar into water and carbon dioxide can occur. Energy that has been trapped by energy-carriers is transported to the respiratory enzyme system for storage in a chemical bonding of phosphorus to molecular carriers. This energy component is known as adenosine triphosphate (ATP) and the energy storage molecule is known as creatine phosphate. Whenever necessary, the body can catalytically clip a phosphate bond off these carriers, releasing as much as 7,000 calories of energy. The energy component, ATP, appears to be the ultimate design of the cellular metabolism of glucose.

When glucose is depleted it is necessary to obtain similar carbon skeletons for ATP production (Fig 1). In shock there is an excellent compensatory mechanism, gluconeogenesis, which transforms the carbon skeleton of amino acids, fatty acids and glycerol to sugar molecules in the energy-producing pathways. It has been said that the amount of glucose available to the body by gluconeogenesis may be almost ten times that derived from glycogen. The

significance of this compensatory mechanism is even more evident
when the limited glycogen stores in the liver and in the muscle
cells are considered.[9]

During injury the neuroendocrine system stimulates the production of emergency energy for vital organ function. The adrenal
cortex produces glucocorticoid hormones which activate gluconeogenesis. Glucocorticoids influence various parts of the glucose
pathway, beginning with the entrance of amino acids such as
alanine into pyruvate, and further stimulate other amino acids to
enter into the tricarboxylic acid (TCA) cycle for the breakdown
of glucose into water, carbon dioxide and energy. A similar mechanism functions when glycerol and fatty acids enter the glucose
pathways through the oxidation of long-chain fatty acids to the
shortened three- or four-carbon fragments and through the entrance of glycerol into the glucose breakdown process. The breakdown of fatty acids can be stimulated by the action of either
epinephrine or glucocorticoids on the enzyme systems, allowing

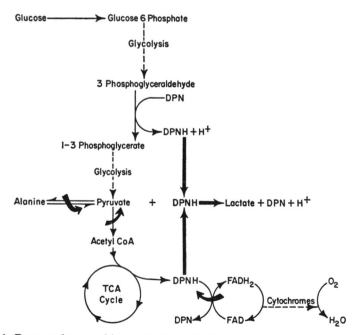

Fig 1. Proposed anaerobic metabolism of glucose in low-flow states.

more glucose to enter the blood stream for energy production in the peripheral tissues.[10, 11]

Without oxygen, only the anaerobic glycolytic cycle can be maintained, limiting glucose metabolism to the pyruvic acid–acetyl coenzyme-A step. Pyruvic acid cannot be oxidized to acetyl–Co-A; therefore, the entrance to the TCA cycle is blocked and pyruvate is then directed toward lactic acid. An increased need for energy stimulates the glycolytic pathway action, augmenting the production of pyruvic acid and thus producing more lactic acid. Most studies have shown that as anoxia increases, the lactic acid content of the serum and cell also increases. The accumulation of lactic acid in peripheral tissues, the incomplete breakdown of fats producing acetone bodies and fatty acids, and the inhibition of amino acid entrance into the energy cycle, dangerously increase the acid load in the blood. This is reflected by a low pH in the blood and tissues, inducing derangements of vital organ metabolism (Fig 2).[12]

If the breakdown of glucose is inhibited there should be a concomitant deficiency in ATP production. An increase in inorganic phosphorus in the liver and kidney due to the catalytic degradation of ATP releasing more phosphorus in the serum has been reported. ATP declines rapidly in the liver, kidney and muscle, and much later in the heart. Since the maintenance of biologic function is dependent on the continuous supply of ATP, its absence causes severe metabolic and physiologic dysfunction in vital organs. Metabolic acidemia combined with ATP depletion is sufficient to cause an irreversible metabolic and, finally, physiologic state.[13]

The effects of corticoids on the cell metabolic pathways have been described by Oji and Shreeve.[14] In radioactive tracer experiments they found that corticoids produced a fivefold increase in the free glucose radioactivity from labeled lactate and malate. We performed similar experiments, giving corticoids to rats in shock, and found a decreased lactate radioactivity and increased labeling of pyruvate and citric acid intermediates, particularly malate. The malate radioactivity may have been due to the entrance of glucose ^{14}C into the dicarboxylic shunt. The shunt reactions are the mechanisms by which citric acid intermediates can be converted into glucose and glycogen. The shunt allows a bypass of the anoxic block of the pyruvate to acetyl–Co-A reactions. Oji and Shreeve

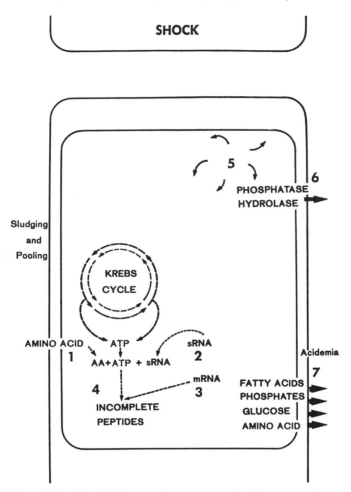

Fig 2. The cell in shock. Decreased energy production at the Krebs cycle limits the activation of amino acids and subsequently depresses protein synthesis. (1) Decreased ATP limits the combining of amino acid and s-RNA. (2) Reduced amount of combined amino acid and s-RNA. (3) m-RNA from the nucleus provides templates for protein synthesis, but (4) end products are not normal; i.e., incomplete peptides (possibly vasoactive) are formed. (5) Lysosome ruptures. (6) Released acid phosphatases and hydrolases escape to the serum. The result is death of the cell. (7) Acidemia.

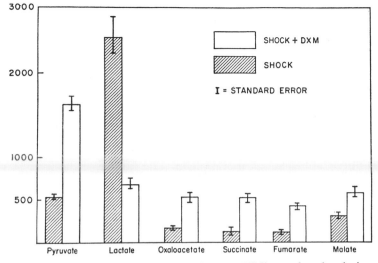

Fig 3. Effect of dexamethasone phosphate (DXM) on the glycolytic and acid intermediates of liver in shock.

also reported an increase of labeled carbon dioxide attributable to a general increase in respiration.

The lactate decrease appears to be corroborated in human studies. We have studied 50 cases of shock in humans, 25 septic and 25 hemorrhagic, and have determined lactate concentrations before and after administration of corticoids. A significant decrease in the lactate concentration was observed after administering pharmacologic doses of corticoids (Fig 3).

Feigelson and Feigelson,[15] working with adrenalectomized rats, reported a decrease of liver ATP without corticoid infusion and an augmented ATP production when corticoids were given. In the human studies, a decrease of serum inorganic phosphate with the use of corticoids indicated further incorporation of phosphate into ATP. This is indirect evidence that corticoids may stimulate ATP formation in the human.

Protein Metabolism

The ability of the carbon skeleton of amino acid to enter the trichloroacetic acid cycle, forming sugar molecules, is the basis for protein breakdown in shock. It is recognized that there is a negative nitrogen balance in shocklike states. This occurs as a result of corticoid-stimulated gluconeogenesis.

Engel,[16] in 1943, demonstrated that hemorrhagic shock in the rat is characterized by rising blood levels of amino nitrogen, mainly because of an increased breakdown of proteins in the peripheral tissues and partly because of the decreased ability of the anoxic liver to metabolize amino acids. He implied, but did not prove, that the depressed rate of deamination of liver amino acids was important in shock metabolism. The failure of the liver to remove amino acids causes decreased urea formation in dogs during hemorrhagic shock. Indeed, the liver dysfunction of animals in severe shock augments the amino acid load of plasma. It is not surprising that infused solutions of amino acids are sometimes poorly tolerated by injured dogs. The liver defect is presumably that of deamination, since the low blood-urea concentrations are not accompanied by ammonia accumulation. This probably is due to the inaction of deamination and transamination enzymes, which depend on oxygen for their function.[17]

Nardi,[18] in 1954, corroborated Engel's work by observing that aminoaciduria accompanies an increased urinary nitrogen excretion in shock. This loss consists of nonessential amino acids normally found in the urine and essential amino acids such as threonine, leucine, isoleucine, lysine and methionine. The reaction to shock is a more active catabolic process than that due to disuse. Definite traces of creatinine and heat-coagulable proteins are excreted during maximum excretion of nitrogen-breakdown molecules. This indicates that the catabolic state is largely produced by the muscle tissue breakdown. Protein catabolism increases blood amino acid levels shortly after shock.

Shock causes disturbances in plasma protein concentrations, in addition to immediate blood-loss effects. Observations in our laboratory and in others have demonstrated that shock was accompanied by a relative increase of the α_2-globulin concentration in plasma.[19] Animals in low-flow states show definite changes in β-globulin concentrations. There is a slight fall in plasma albumin, combined with a rise in globulin fraction and fibrinogen. The α_2-

globulin increase has been postulated to reside in a glycoprotein fraction, particularly the seromucoid. In our shock experiments, seromucoids increased threefold when compared to the normal. These increases are attributed to the haptoglobulin or antitrypsin macromolecules fixing the destroyed red blood cell and proteolytic enzymes. The enzymes may be a result of necrosis.[20]

Apparently, muscle is the major source of excessive excretion of nitrogen, sulfur, phosphorus, potassium, and creatinine in the urine.[21-23]

The effect of corticoids on protein metabolism was discussed previously. Corticoids induce enzyme biosynthesis, thus promoting gluconeogenesis.

Fat Metabolism

Lipolysis, or breakdown of fat tissue, is initiated by the catecholamines, epinephrine, norepinephrine and glucocorticoids. It has been demonstrated experimentally that this process is due to the accelerated breakdown of triglycerides to free fatty acids. The emergency mechanism responsible for the initiation of fat breakdown is a well-functioning adrenal cortex.[24, 25] Glucocorticoids may directly stimulate release of free fatty acids. Thyroid hormone also plays a significant role, as evidenced by various responses of adrenergic agents on release of free fatty acid with and without thyroid hormone. Once released, fatty acids are then utilized in the energy-producing cycles previously described.

The rapid mobilization of fats during stress or corticoid infusion is vitally important to the patient, since the calorific values of fats are much greater than those of glucose and protein. Fats approach a theoretical yield of nine calories per gram, while carbohydrates and proteins produce only four calories per gram. However, the use of fatty acids for ATP production has the inherent danger of acidosis. Under stress the metabolic degradation of fats yields considerable quantities of acetone and ketone bodies, aceto-acetic acid, and β-hydroxy-butyric acid. These molecules may be considered normal by-products of the oxidation of fatty acids; they are produced in small quantities during normal metabolism. When shock occurs, carbohydrate utilization is deficient; the energy requirements of the body must be met by the use of more fats, and greater production of ketones in the liver may exceed the ability of that organ to accomplish complete oxidation. Consequently, ketones overflow into the blood and are excreted in the urine. Peripheral tissues metabolize ketones for energy but cannot cope with an overload of these fat metabolites. Because of the marked constriction of peripheral tissues and the absence of oxygen in shock, ketone oxidation deteriorates. Concomitantly, poor perfusion through the liver decreases fatty acid oxidation. This metabolic acidemia is compounded by the production of lactate and by aminoaciduria due to anoxia.[26-28]

Electrolyte Metabolism

Study of the serum electrolyte changes in patients undergoing various degrees of hemorrhage in operative trauma was performed by the Hahnemann group.[29] Hourly studies were performed during surgery and for several hours postoperatively, particularly on those patients who were refractory to shock therapy. Electrolyte changes were correlated with changes in electrocardiograms. A predictable rise in the concentration of phosphate in the blood was found in 100 patients. There was a fall in sodium concentration and a rise in potassium. Occasionally a patient exhibited a sharp drop in the concentration of calcium. Correlation of the fall of calcium to the electrocardiographic findings demonstrated its relationship to marked tachycardia. Several patients responded dramatically to intravenous infusions of calcium gluconate after blood pressure had failed to respond to adequate transfusion.[30,21,31]

The role of potassium in shock is fundamental. Shock depletes the energy component ATP, impairing the cell membrane pump function and resulting in a loss of intracellular potassium to the extracellular compartment. This is further complicated by metabolic acidemia supporting hyperkalemia. The increased potassium concentrations can be fatal and may directly influence the development of cardiac standstill in patients in shock. This is corroborated by the sensitivity to potassium administration exhibited by animals in shock.

Potassium has a specific effect on protein synthesis, which is postulated to be at the step where the amino acid enters the polypeptide chain. Low intracellular potassium will therefore have an effect on the production of immunoproteins in the lymphocyte. This is deleterious to septic shock patients who need antibodies to combat toxins. Intracellularly, the main role of potassium is the buffering or neutralizing of the phosphate ester. Phosphate metabolism is intimately associated with the development of the energy component ATP. Therefore, potassium depletion has a profound effect on the previously impaired energy pathways.

Giving potassium without glucose to a patient in shock can be dangerous; however, with a vehicle of high concentrations of glucose and adequate doses of insulin, the potassium will be rerouted intracellularly, repairing the metabolic deficit.

In shock there are three salient and interdependent factors: fluid loss, sodium loss, and potassium liberation. Singly, these factors can be detrimental; their concerted action is fatal. Because of the loss of ATP, there is functional impairment of the sodium-potassium pump, causing the cellular edema of energy depletion. A basic pathologic finding is the accumulation of fluids in traumatized cells. This in uninhibited by osmotic solutions and replacement therapy is sufficient only when it effects maximum swelling of the tissues and corrects the depletion of fluids, electrolytes and proteins.[29,32,33,34]

An investigation of the wounded in the Korean Conflict showed a 100% magnesium increase in the serum, indicative of magnesium exudation from traumatized tissue or the body's attempt to use cationic magnesium to combat metabolic acidemia.[35]

Studies by Moyer and associates,[29] and Shires et al.[33,34] suggested that in shock states there is a shift of water from the extracellular to the intracellular compartments. Glucocorticoids have been reported to reverse this shift. This has been especially apparent in therapy of intracellular cerebral edema. However, the glucocorticoid role in water homeostasis restoration has not been established. Corticoids have also been reported to stabilize plasma membranes, especially the vascular and endothelial cells. This would reverse the endothelial permeability in the anoxic state of shock.

CORRELATION OF ULTRAMICROSCOPIC PATHOLOGY AND BIOCHEMISTRY

A fascinating aspect of the metabolic concept of shock is the correlation of the locus of biochemical function and the pathologic lesion seen with the ultramicroscope. Cellular energy production involves several cell organelles: the ergastoplasm or cytoplasm, the mitochondria, the microsomes, the lysosomes, and the endoplasmic reticulum. The energy pathways flux through the cell in the following manner: Glucose and potassium are absorbed by the energy-fueled cell membrane pump. The cell membrane pump is stimulated by insulin. Glucose is then converted to glucose-6-phosphate and may be synthesized to glycogen for storage in the cytoplasm. Glycogen and glucose-6-phosphate can be degraded to trioses in the anaerobic glycolytic cycle located in the cytoplasm. Aerobic oxidation of trioses (Krebs cycle) occurs in the mitochondria. The oxidation of the Krebs cycle intermediates produces energy which is trapped by coenzyme carriers (nicotinamide adenine dinucleotide). These allow entrance to the respiratory cycle in the mitochondrial cristae. The respiratory cycle produces ATP. ATP is secreted in the cytoplasm and may activate amino acids which have been selectively absorbed by the cell membrane. Activated amino acids are transferred to soluble ribonucleic acid (RNA) for transport to the ribosomes in the endoplasmic reticulum. DNA-dependent messenger-RNA induces the production of the specific proteins, immunoproteins, collagen and enzyme systems. In ATP depletion these proteins are not produced. This deficit is particularly significant in septic shock, when antibody formation is depressed. ATP also sustains the cell membrane pump function by maintaining potassium intracellularly and sodium extracellularly. Disruption of this function allows an influx of sodium and water into the cell, specifically in the mitochondria. Ultramicroscopic studies of the cell have shown that in profound shock the endoplasmic reticulum is disrupted, protoplasmic and mitochondrial edema are present, and there is cell lysis, which probably is due to lysosomal membrane rupture. The lysosomes contain the lytic enzymes and since the lysosome membrane is sensitive to pH changes, marked intracellular acidosis causes the membrane to burst, secreting lytic enzymes. Necrosis and autolysis ensue.[36,37]

Recent observations have focused attention on the possibility that some of the glucocorticoid effects on the tissue may be due to their ability to stabilize lysosomal membranes. Lysosome subcellular particles are surrounded by a lipoprotein membrane which is disrupted in various ways (ischemia, endotoxin, ultraviolet irradiation, streptolysin and hypervitaminosis A), releasing lytic enzymes. Corticoids appear to prevent membrane rupture, thereby suppressing acid hydrolase release, an effect which has been noted in several tissues including bone, gastrointestinal mucosa, cartilage, and liver. Janoff[38] reported that in shock, corticoids protect the lysosomal membranes.

THERAPEUTIC CONCEPTS

The following therapeutic concepts have been derived from these cellular studies:

Reparation of the damaged biochemical mechanism should be an integral aspect of the therapeutic concept of shock. The main metabolic acid load is decreased by the treatment of acid-base changes and by the stimulation of enzyme systems, reversing lactic acid to intermediates in the glycolytic metabolic pathways. Corticoids protect the lysosomal membrane against pH changes. In our laboratories, decreases in lactic acidemia, aminoacidemia and hyperphosphatemia of shock have been noted after corticoid administration (Figs 4 and 5). Therefore, the following concept evolved: Corticoids induce gluconeogenesis, converting the amino acid carbon skeletons to energy-producing trioses or citric acid intermediates. This generates the citric acid cycle, yielding more ATP. When more ATP is produced there is an increased utilization of free phosphates. Besides these molecular changes, corticoids augment tissue perfusion by capillary vasodilation. This improves oxygen and micronutrient uptake.[39]

Present studies indicate that shock is a molecular disease having its basic defect in the energy-formation pathways of the cell. The use of corticoids in low-flow states is one of the initial attempts at treating these conditions on a molecular level. The investigative evidence suggests that these hormones have a stimulatory, salutary effect on cell metabolism in the shock state.

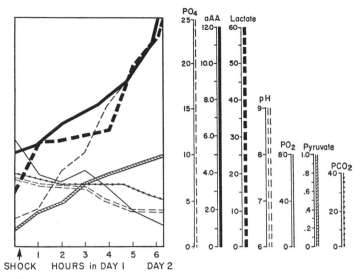

Fig 4. Biochemical parameters in shock.

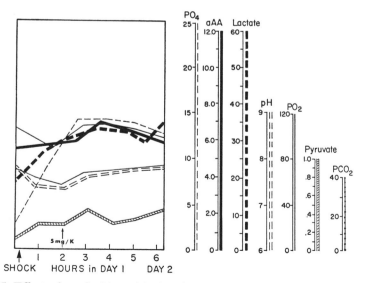

Fig 5. Effect of corticoids on biochemical parameters in shock.

REFERENCES

1. Hench, P. S., Kendall, E. C., Slocumb, C. H., and Polley, H. F.: The Effect of a Hormone of the Adrenal Cortex (17-Hydroxy-11-Dehydro-corticosterone: Compound E) and of Pituitary Adrenocorticotropic Hormone on Rheumatoid Arthritis, *Proc. Mayo Clin.* **24**:181, 1949.

2. Melby, J. C., Egdahl, R. H., and Spink, W. W.: Effect of *Brucella* Endotoxin on Adrenocortical Function in the Dog, *Fed. Proc.* **16**:425, 1957.

3. Lillehei, R. C., Longerbeam, J. K., Bloch, J. H., and Manax, W. G.: The Nature of Irreversible Shock; Experimental and Clinical Observations, *Ann. Surg.* **160**:682, 1964.

4. Sullivan, T. J., and Cavanagh, D.: Corticosteroids in Endotoxin Shock, *Arch. Surg.* **92**:732–739 (May), 1966.

5. Weil, M. H.: The Cardiovascular Effects of Corticosteroids, *Circulation* **25**:718, 1962.

6. Fine, J., *et al.*: New Developments in Therapy of Refractory Traumatic Shock, *Arch. Surg.* **96**:163–175 (Feb.), 1968.

7. Page, I. H.: "Some Neurohumoral and Endocrine Aspects of Shock," in Seeley, S. F., and Weisiger, J. R. (eds.): *Proceedings of a Conference on Recent Progress and Present Problems in the Field of Shock. Fed. Proc.* **20**:75, 1961.

8. Youmans, P. L., Green, H. D., and Denison, A. B., Jr.: Nature of the Vasodilator and Vasoconstrictor Receptors in Skeletal Muscle of the Dog, *Circulation Res.* **3**:171, 1955.

9. Green, H. D., and Rapela, C. E.: "Neurogenic and Autoregulation of the Resistance and Capacitance Components of the Peripheral Vascular System" in Mills, L. C., and Moyer, J. H. (eds.): *Shock and Hypotension* (New York: Grune & Stratton, Inc., 1965), pp. 91–110.

10. Levenson, S. M., Eiheber, A., and Malm, O. J.: "Nutritional and Metabolic Aspects of Shock," in Seeley, S. F., and Weisiger, J. R. (eds.): *Proceedings of a Conference of Recent Progress and Present Problems in the Field of Shock. Fed. Proc.* **20**:99, 1961.

11. Migone, L.: "Metabolic Aspects of Shock," in Bock, K. D. (ed.): *Pathogenesis and Therapy: An International Symposium* (New York: Academic Press, Inc., 1962), pp. 76–79.

12. Schumer, W.: Lactic Acid as a Factor in the Production of Irreversibility in Oligohemic Shock, *Nature* **212**:1210, 1967.

13. Tremolières, J., and Dérache, R.: "Métabolisme des composes phosphores et spécialement des nucléotides dans le tissu traumatisé," in Stoner, H. B., and Threlfall, C. J. (eds.): *The Biochemical Response in Injury* (Springfield, Ill.: Charles C Thomas Publisher, 1960), pp. 23–50.

14. Oji, N., and Shreeve, W. W.: Gluconeogenesis from C^{14}- and 3H-Labeled Substrates in Normal and Cortisone-Treated Rats, *Endocrinology* **78**:765, 1966.

15. Feigelson, P., and Feigelson, M.: "Studies on the Mechanism of Cortisone Actions," in Litweck, G., and Kritchewsky, D. (eds.): *Actions*

of Hormones on Molecular Processes (Evanston, Ill.: J. Wiley & Sons, Inc., 1964), pp. 218–233.

16. Engel, F. L.: The Significance of the Metabolic Changes During Shock, *Ann. New York Acad. Sc.* **55**:381, 1952.

17. Fleck, A., and Munro, H. N.: Protein Metabolism After Injury, *Metabolism* **12**:783, 1963.

18. Nardi, J. L.: "Essential and Nonessential" Amino Acids in Urine of Severely Burned Patients, *J. Clin. Invest.* **33**:847, 1954.

19. Harper, H. A.: *Review of Physiological Chemistry* (Los Altos, Calif.: Lange Medical Publications, 1963), p. 437.

20. Kukral, J. C., Pancner, R. J., Louch, J., and Winzler, R. J.: Synthesis of Canine Seromucoid Before and After Total Hepatectomy, *Amer. J. Physiol.* **202**:1087, 1962.

21. Millican, R. C.: "Plasma Protein Distribution Studies in Traumatic Shock," in Mills, L. C., and Moyer, J. H. (eds.): *Shock and Hypotension, Pathogenesis and Treatment* (New York: Grune & Stratton, Inc., 1965), pp. 351–359.

22. Schumer, W.: Production of Seromucoid Protein Fraction by Low-Flow States, *Surg. Forum* **16**:13, 1965.

23. Shetlar, M. R.: Serum Glycoproteins: Their Origin and Significance, *Ann. New York Acad. Sc.* **94**:44, 1961.

24. Klausner, H., and Heimberg, M.: Effect of Adrenocortical Hormones on Release of Triglycerides and Glucose by Liver, *Amer. J. Physiol.* **212**:1236, 1967.

25. Renold, A. E., Cahill, G. F., Jr., Leboeuf, B., and Herrera, M. G.: "Effect of Adrenal Hormones Upon Adipose Tissue," in Wolstenholme, G. E. W., and O'Connor, M. (eds.): *Metabolic Effects of Adrenal Hormones*. Ciba Foundation Study Group No. 6 (Boston: Little, Brown & Company, 1960), pp. 68–81.

26. Masoro, E. J.: "The Effect of Physical Injury on Lipid Metabolism" in Stoner, H. B., and Threlfall, C. J. (eds.): *The Biochemical Response to Injury. A Symposium* (Springfield, Ill.: Charles C Thomas, Publisher, 1960), p. 467.

27. Rodahl, K., and Issekutz, B. (eds.): *Fat as a Tissue* (New York: McGraw-Hill Book Company, Inc., 1964), p. 428.

28. Schumer, W.: Metabolism of the Fat Cell in Low-Flow States, *J. Surg. Res.* **6**:254, 1966.

29. Moyer, C. A., Margraf, H. W., and Monafo, W. W., Jr.: Burn Shock and Extravascular Sodium Deficiency: Treatment with Ringer's Solution with Lactate, *Arch. Surg.* **90**:799, 1965.

30. Fuhrman, F. A., and Crismon, J. M.: Muscle Electrolytes in Rats Following Ischemia Produced by Tourniquet, *Amer. J. Physiol.* **167**:289, 1951.

31. Millican, R. C.: Tourniquet Shock in Mice: Na^{22} and S^{35} Plasma Turnover in the Accumulated Fluid in Area of Injury, *Amer. J. Physiol.* **179**:529, 1954.

32. Coleman, B., and Glaviano, V. V.: Electrolyte and Water Distribution

in the Heart in Irreversible Hemorrhagic Shock, *Amer. J. Physiol.* **207**: 352, 1964.

33. Shires, T., and Carrico, C. J.: *Current Status of the Shock Problems: Current Problems in Surgery* (Chicago: Year Book Medical Publishers, Inc., 1966), p. 67.

34. Shires, T., Colin, D., Carrico, J., and Lightfoot, S.: Fluid Therapy in Hemorrhagic Shock, *Arch. Surg.* **88**:688, 1964.

35. Aikawa, J. D.: *The Role of Magnesium in Biologic Process* (Springfield, Ill.: Charles C Thomas, Publisher, 1963), p. 117.

36. Holden, W. D., DePalma, R. G., Drucker, W. R., and McKalen, A.: Ultrastructural Changes in Hemorrhagic Shock: Electron Microscopic Study of Liver, Kidney and Striated Muscle Cells in Rats, *Ann. Surg.* **162**: 517, 1965.

37. Martin, A. M., and Hackel, D. B.: An Electron Microscopic Study of the Progression of Myocardial Lesions in the Dog After Hemorrhagic Shock, *Lab. Invest.* **15**:243, 1966.

38. Janoff, A., Weissman, G., Zweifach, B. W., and Thomas, L.: Pathogenesis of Experimental Shock. IV. Studies on Lysosomes in Normal and Tolerant Animals Subjected to Lethal Trauma and Endotoxemia, *J. Exp. Med.* **116**:451, 1962.

39. Schumer, W.: Physiochemical Effect of Dexamethasone on the Primate in Oligemic Shock, *Arch. Surg.* **98**:259–261, 1969.

Therapy of Shock
with Corticosteroids

Hemorrhagic Shock

MAX H. WEIL, M.D., Ph.D.

When a potent antibiotic tetracycline was first used to treat brucellosis, the drug sometimes produced a condition simulating the shock state. Not unlike the Herxheimer reaction which occurs during treatment of syphillis, it might have been regarded simply as part of the natural course of the disease under treatment. However, Spink and Braude,[1] who originally observed this phenomenon, wondered what it really represented. In the next several years, the investigators who were to come from the laboratories of these outstanding workers were to clarify the mechanism of this shock-like phenomenon and call attention to its important medical implications. Spink and Anderson[2] in 1951 were the first to describe the role of corticosteroids in preventing the lethal effects of bacterial endotoxin. Later, I had the good personal fortune to begin my investigative career in Dr. Spink's laboratory, and to share in the further investigation of this subject.

In 1955, we recognized some striking similarities between the immediate reaction to intravenous injection of bacterial endotoxin and the typical anaphylactic reaction.[3] The anaphylactoid reaction produced by endotoxin, like the anaphylactic reaction, precipitates a complex series of hemodynamic, metabolic, and hematologic events. These, in turn, are modified by a host of pharmacologic agents, including adrenergic, antihistaminic, anesthetic, and corticoid drugs. Endotoxin, like the antigen-antibody reaction, triggers a reaction in plasma. The white cell component of plasma appears to be an important intermediary to this reaction which, as observed in the dog, includes systemic arterial hypotension, portal and pulmonary hypertension, leukopenia, thrombocytopenia, intravascular coagulation, a pronounced increase in circulating epinephrine, glucocorticoid, histamine, and characteristic pathological changes in the splanchnic organs.[3,4]

Large doses of glucocorticoids which had prevented the fatal reaction of mice to endotoxin were also effective in decreasing mortality in rats[5] and the severity of the reaction in dogs.[6] After the efficacy of glucocorticoid in modifying the lethal effects of endotoxin had been demonstrated, we investigated pharmacologic aspects of this subject, especially with regard to differences in the effectiveness of various glucocorticoid analogues. Before I left Dr. Spink's laboratory I had observed the work of his colleague, Dr. J. C. Melby,[7] who clearly established that cortisol secretion was maximal after endotoxin had produced shock, and that the therapeutic value of steroid treatment was due to a drug effect rather than hormonal replacement. The purpose of our work in the late 1950's was to provide objective guidelines by which this drug could be used with maximal efficacy but minimal toxicity.[8] The practical implication of this work had become even more significant after Lillehei and MacLean[9] recommended the routine use of hydrocortisone for various types of shock, in even larger doses than had previously been used.

MATERIALS AND METHODS

Endotoxin

A model in which Swiss-Webster mice received a lethal dose of *E. coli* endotoxin by intraperitoneal injection was first used.

The striking therapeutic efficacy of synthetic corticosteroid analogues could not be achieved with cortisol succinate or cortisol phosphate. Lethal effects attributable to the high dose of steroid appeared before the maximally effective dose could be given. In the case of methylprednisolone, the therapeutic effect was achieved before drug toxicity was manifested. Subsequently, with dexamethasone (and also triamcinolone) we were able to show more than a fortyfold separation between the toxic and therapeutic doses. This suggested that the toxicity, in this mouse system, was independent of glucocorticoid potency but closely related to the amount of drug (by weight) administered to the animals, by the intraperitoneal route (Table).

TABLE. Toxic-Therapeutic Ratios of Glucocorticoids

	Therapeutic LD_{50}/ED_{50}	Max. Effectiveness LD_{01}/ED_{50}
Dexamethasone phosphate	282	45
Methylprednisolone succinate	45	2
Prednisolone phosphate	36	6
Cortisol succinate	17	$<<1$
Cortisol phosphate	30	$<<1$

Ratio of toxic therapeutic doses of glucocorticoid in mg/kg:

LD_{50} = lethal dose for 50 per cent

ED_{50} = effective (survival) dose for 50 per cent

LD_{01} = lethal dose for 1 per cent

Hemodynamic Actions

After the University of Southern California Shock Ward had been established at the Los Angeles County General Hospital, we were able to accumulate data on patients. We found that when large doses of glucocorticoids were administered to patients in bacterial shock, there was a predictable increase in cardiac output over a period of between one-half hour and two hours, and a fall in peripheral arterial resistance[10] (Fig 1). Lillehei[11] at the same time described effects he had observed during studies on blood flow through the mesenteric circuit: that effects of corticosteroids were in some ways similar to those of alpha-adrenergic-blocking drugs.

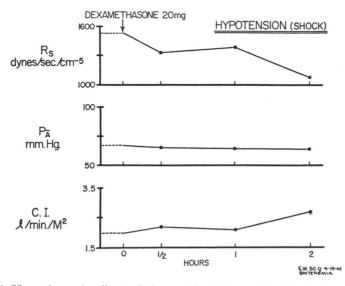

Fig 1. Hemodynamic effects of glucocorticoid in a patient in shock.

From: Sambhi, M. P., Weil, M. H., and Udhoji, V. N.: Acute Pharmacodynamic Effects of Glucocorticoids: Cardiac Output and Related Hemodynamic Changes in Normal Subjects and Patients in Shock, *Circulation* **31**: 523-530, 1965. By permission of the American Heart Association, Inc.

Hemorrhagic Shock

Armed with this preliminary information, we looked for another test system with which we could study effects of corticosteroid drugs on hemorrhagic shock, preferably in a small animal species. A technique was developed in which hemorrhagic shock was produced under controlled conditions in the Wistar rat. Since as many as four animals were included in a single experiment, the statistical significance of the data was greatly increased. The investment of time and effort in a single experiment was admittedly great, but it was justified because fewer experiments were needed. The femoral artery was cannulated for pressure recording and bleeding and a femoral vein was cannulated for the purpose of injection of the drugs. The methods have been described in detail elsewhere.[12]

Pressure in a reservoir connected to the arterial cannula was reduced and maintained at this level for 240 minutes. The blood was then reinfused. Bleeding was mechanically slowed by the high resistance of the small catheter inserted into the artery. At the end of the bleeding periods, the pressure in the reservoirs was increased and blood was thereby reinfused into the rats. During bleeding, a consistent but unexpected finding was that the heart rate decreased rather than increased as arterial pressure declined. The respiratory rate also decreased rather than increased. The hematocrit decreased, evidence of hemodilution during the interval of bleeding. A fall in oxygen consumption, a decline in blood pH (indicative of metabolic acidosis) and a relatively smaller decline in PCO_2 were observed over the 240-minute period. A progressive increase in blood lactate was measured and this was the metabolic consequence of an oxygen deficit. Incidentally, we found that pyruvate contributed no additional information which was not inherent in measurement of lactate alone. The computation of excess lactate and lactate/pyruvate did not increase the predictability of oxygen deficit.[13]

When animals were treated with corticosteroid or aldosterone at the end of the 240-minute bleeding period, survival was significantly increased in comparison to controls.[14] However, there were differences in survival among animals treated with hydrocortisone (300 mg/kg) or equivalent amounts of methylprednisolone (40 mg/kg) or dexamethasone (8 mg/kg). The best results were obtained with dexamethasone, although in this rat experiment the differences between dexamethasone and cortisol were not statistically significant. With methylprednisolone, survival rate was somewhat lower. A measure of animal responsiveness in the 16 hours following reinfusion demonstrated early resuscitation of treated animals in comparison to untreated controls (Fig 2).

Aldosterone also increased survival, but a critical level of dosage was identified. After animals received more than 0.4 mg/kg of aldosterone, the survival rate fell off sharply. The best dose was 0.2 mg/kg. However, even at the optimal dose, aldosterone proved less effective than glucocorticoid in increasing survival (Fig 3).

When the metabolic function of animals was measured in a metabolic chamber, a significantly greater oxygen consumption was observed after treatment with dexamethasone. Concomitantly an increase in pH to levels intermediate between the nonhemorrhage controls and the bled, untreated animals, was observed,

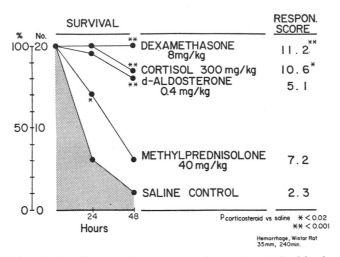

Fig 2.† Survival and responsiveness score in rats treated with glucocorticoids at the time of reinfusion after 240 minutes of bleeding.

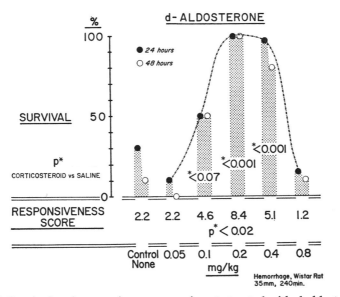

Fig 3.† Survival and responsiveness score in rats treated with d-aldosterone at the time of reinfusion of blood after 240 minutes of bleeding.

† Figures 2 and 3 are Figs 3 and 4 respectively from: Weil, M. H., and Whigham, H.: Corticosteroids for Reversal of Hemorrhagic Shock in Rats, *Amer. J. Physiol.* **209**: 815-818 (October), 1965.

demonstrating that the increased survival was associated with an increase in oxygen consumption and lesser severity of metabolic (anoxic) acidosis.

RATIONALE OF CORTICOSTEROID TREATMENT

Some years ago, Guyton and Crowell indicated the critical nature of oxygen debt in explaining the survival of animals (dogs) in hemorrhagic shock.[15] The critical oxygen debt or oxygen deficit is the issue which determines survival. The predictability of survival, both in experimental animals and in patients on the basis of lactate excess, reflects the same phenomenon.[16] When corticosteroids are used to increase blood flow, oxygen delivery is improved. This, in turn, accounts for the improvement in pH, the lessened metabolic acidosis, the increased early responsiveness and the increase in survival after otherwise fatal hemorrhage.

SUMMARY AND CONCLUSIONS

Glucocorticoids under experimental conditions prevent fatal circulatory failure after hemorrhage as they do after shock produced by injection of endotoxin. Differences in effectiveness of various glucocorticoid analogues have been identified. In experimental models, the very large doses of glucocorticoid required for maximal efficacy result in drug toxicity. Since the toxic effects in mice are directly related not to glucocorticoid potency, but to the physical weight of the drug injected, the better results consistently observed with dexamethasone are probably explained by its higher glucocorticoid potency on a weight basis.

There are important species differences in adrenal metabolism and we would not suggest direct application of the present observations, based largely on studies in mice and rats, to treatment of human patients. However, the increases in effective blood flow and oxygen consumption, the decrease in oxygen deficit and lactate, and greater survival rate after therapy with glucocorticoid are consistent with hemodynamic effects observed in patients. Still needed is an objective study in patients to confirm not only the effectiveness of glucocorticoids, but to assure that their use for routine treatment of hemorrhagic shock does not entail special hazards that may of themselves preclude their routine employment.

REFERENCES

1. Spink, W. W., Braude, A. I., Castaneda, M. R., and Silva Goytia, R.: Aureomycin Therapy in Human Brucellosis Due to *Brucella melitensis, JAMA* **138**:1145–1148, 1948.
2. Spink, W. W., and Anderson, D.: Studies Relating to Differential Diagnosis of Brucellosis and Infectious Mononucleosis: Clinical, Hematologic, and Serologic Observations, *Tr. A. Amer. Physicians* **64**:428–434, 1951.
3. Weil, M. H., and Spink, W. W.: A Comparison of Shock Due to Endotoxin with Anaphylactic Shock, *J. Lab. Clin. Med.* **50**:501–515, 1957.
4. Hinshaw, L. B., Kuida, H., Gilbert, R. P., and Visscher, M. B.: Influence of Perfusate Characteristics on Pulmonary Vascular Response to Endotoxin, *Amer. J. Physiol.* **191**:293–295, 1957.
5. Weil, M. H.: Endotoxin Shock, *Clin. Obstet. Gynec.* **4**:971–983, 1961.
6. Weil, M. H., and Miller, B. S.: Experimental Studies on Therapy of Circulatory Failure Produced by Endotoxin, *J. Lab. Clin. Med.* **57**:683–693, 1961.
7. Melby, J. C., and Spink, W. W.: Comparative Studies on Adrenal Cortical Function and Cortisol Metabolism in Healthy Adults and in Patients with Shock Due to Infection, *J. Clin. Invest.* **37**:1791–1798, 1958.
8. Weil, M. H., and Allen, K. S.: Adrenocortical Steroid for Therapy of Acute Hypotension: Special Reference to Experiments on Shock Produced by Endotoxin, *Amer. Pract. Digest Treat.* **12**:162–168, 1961.
9. Lillehei, R. C., and MacLean, L. D.: Physiological Approach to Successful Treatment of Endotoxin Shock in the Experimental Animal, *Arch. Surg.* **78**:464–471, 1959.
10. Sambhi, M. P., Weil, M. H., and Udhoji, V. N.: Acute Pharmacodynamic Effects of Glucocorticoids: Cardiac Output and Related Hemodynamic Changes in Normal Subjects and Patients in Shock, *Circulation* **31**:523–530, 1965.
11. Lillehei, R. C., Longerbeam, J. K., and Rosenberg, J. C.: The Nature of Irreversible Shock: Its Relationship to Intestinal Changes. In *Shock: Pathogenesis and Therapy*; An International Symposium, Stockholm, 27th–30th June, 1961. K. D. Bock, ed. (Berlin: Springer, 1962).
12. Weil, M. H., and Whigham, H.: Corticosteroids for Reversal of Hemorrhagic Shock in Rats, *Amer. J. Physiol.* **209**:815–818, 1965.
13. Weil, M. H., Afifi, A. A., Whigham, W., and Marbach, E. P.: Blood Lactate and Pyruvate for Assessing the Severity of Acute Circulatory Failure (Shock), *Circulation* **35**: (suppl. II) 264–265, 1967.

14. Whigham, H., and Weil, M. H.: A Model for the Study of Hemorrhagic Shock in the Rat: Development of the Method, *J. Applied Physiol.* **21**:1860–1863, 1966.

15. Guyton, A. C., and Crowell, J. W.: Dynamics of the Heart in Shock, *Fed. Proc.* **20**: (suppl. 9) 55, 1961.

16. Broder, G., and Weil, M. H.: Excess Lactate: An Index of Reversibility of Shock in Human Patients, *Science* **143**:1457–1459, 1964.

Endotoxin Shock

WESLEY W. SPINK, M.D.

In 1954, Spink and Anderson[1] reported that pretreatment with cortisone protected mice against lethal doses of endotoxin. This was contrary to the observations of others[2] who, in the same type of experiment, described the lesions of a generalized and fatal Shwartzman reaction in rabbits. In subsequent investigations, dogs were protected with corticosteroids, and we could never demonstrate the Shwartzman reaction in this species. The Shwartzman phenomenon in conjunction with steroid and endotoxin usually occurs in rabbits, but a similar reaction is also observed in man or other animal species. Of considerable importance clinically were studies on canine endotoxin shock in which cortisol administered *after* the onset of shock did not afford protection.[3] However, the simultaneous use of cortisol and a vasopressor (metaraminol) resulted in higher survival rates, although this result did not occur when either agent was used alone.

This study was supported by USPHS Research Grant AI 04415–06 from the National Institutes of Health.

CLINICAL EXPERIENCE

Before discussing corticosteroid therapy in human endotoxin shock, I should like to describe our general experience at the University of Minnesota Medical Center with sepsis due to gram-negative organisms. Between 1950 and 1955, there were 278 patients with bacteremia due to gram-negative bacilli, of which 43 manifested shock, with a mortality of 65%.[4] During the latter part of this period, therapy for shock included corticosteroid and metaraminol. Although the results were encouraging, a definitive evaluation of this combination required more data.

Clinical Data Analysis

To obtain more precise information on bacteremia and on endotoxin shock, Dr. Herbert DuPont and I analyzed data on 892 patients with bacteremia at the University of Minnesota Medical Center between 1958 and 1966. Important data in the evaluation of therapy in bacteremia with and without shock include general host factors, such as the underlying state of health prior to the onset of bacteremia. The outlook for a healthy young woman who develops bacteremia with shock in the postpartum period is far superior to that for an aged person with degenerative disease and malignancy who acquires bacteremia and shock immediately after extensive surgery and while receiving immunosuppressive drugs. This is shown in Table I, in which such factors

TABLE I. RELATIONS OF GENERAL HOST FACTORS TO MORTALITY IN 892 CASES OF GRAM-NEGATIVE BACTEREMIA

Good Prognosis			Intermediate			Poor Prognosis		
No.	Deaths	(%)	No.	Deaths	(%)	No.	Deaths	(%)
371	67	(18)	369	240	(65)	152	131	(86)

were evaluated prior to the development of bacteremia. The group in whom bacteremia developed while they were otherwise in a state of good health had a mortality of 18%, whereas 86% of those in precarious health died. The evaluation of therapy in human endotoxin shock requires more of this kind of data.

Bacterial Identification

Another major factor in the outcome for the patient is the identification of the specific bacteria invading the bloodstream (Table II). In line with the findings of other investigators, we

TABLE II. INCIDENCE OF GRAM-NEGATIVE ORGANISMS CAUSING BACTEREMIA IN 892 PATIENTS

Escherichia coli	244	Flavobacterium	17
Kleb.-Enterobact.-Serratia	165	Salmonella	11
Pseudomonas	103	Herellea and Mima	8
Proteus	72	Alkaligenes	6
Bacteroides	45	Miscellaneous	12
H. influenzae	31	"Multiple"	178

found that *Escherichia coli* is the most common offender. The second most common cause of bacteremia is the *Klebsiella-Enterobacter-Serratia* group. Then follow the species of *Pseudomonas* and *Proteus*. Such information has significant prognostic meaning in the selection of the proper antibiotic or antibiotics early in the course of the bacteremia. It is significant that there were more than a hundred cases with "multiple" species; that is, more than one species was recovered from a blood culture. This finding indicates a poor prognosis, and usually suggests a seriously compromised defense mechanism against microbial invasion.

Choice of Antibiotic

The prompt identification of the causative agent or agents in a bloodstream infection augurs well for the patient, provided the proper antimicrobial drug or drugs is selected. In Table III are presented the results of antibiotic treatment in 501 cases of

TABLE III. RESULTS IN 501 PATIENTS WITH GRAM-NEGATIVE BACTEREMIA WITH AND WITHOUT ANTIBIOTIC THERAPY

	Number	Died	(%)
No treatment	92	74	(80)
Penicillin	48	37	(77)
Coly-Mycin, Polymyxin	101	60	(59)
Kanamycin	35	14	(40)
Chloramphenicol, Penicillin	109	37	(34)
Tetracycline, Penicillin	116	37	(32)

bacteremia due to gram-negative organisms. The mortality in patients receiving no treatment was 80%, due principally to the fact that bacteriologic findings were not known before death. The mortality was essentially the same (70%) in those receiving only penicillin. Most of the patients receiving colistimethate or polymyxin had bacteremia due to *Pseudomonas*. An encouraging, but not entirely optimistic, aspect was a mortality of 40% in patients having one of the *Klebsiella-Enterobacter-Serratia* group in the bloodstream. It was in the latter group, especially, that precise *in vitro* sensitivity tests were carried out in order to select the most appropriate drug. The mortality in patients receiving either chloramphenicol and penicillin, or tetracycline and penicillin, was essentially the same (34% and 32%, respectively). The chloramphenicol-penicillin combination was used most commonly for infections due to the *Proteus* species, and the tetracycline-penicillin for *E. coli*.

Bacteremia vs. Septic Shock

Of the 892 patients with bacteremia due to gram-negative organisms, 274 (31%) had evidence of endotoxin shock. The main findings were hypotension and oliguria. A protocol of drug therapy carried out in the majority of the patients in this study included a pressor drug, usually metaraminol, and cortisol. Toward the end of the study, larger pharmacologic doses of cortisol were used, a minimum of 50 mg/kg as soon as possible, as recommended by Dr. Richard Lillehei, a surgical colleague.

Steroid Therapy

Patients not receiving a vasopressor drug or steroid had a mortality of 70% (Table IV). Such therapy was in many cases not provided, because the nature of the shock was not clear; that is, shock occurred terminally, or bacteriologic data were not available when shock developed. The mortality was 85% in those receiving only steroid. Those given a vasopressor drug, usually metaraminol, and a low dose of steroid had a mortality of 87%. The most encouraging result, reflecting a trend of recent years, was a mortality of 59% in those receiving a vasopressor drug and

TABLE IV. RELATION OF TREATMENT TO OUTCOME IN 274 PATIENTS
WITH ENDOTOXIN SHOCK

| | Steroid Therapy | | | | | | | |
| | No Steroid | | | Low Dosage | | | High Dosage | | |
Vasoactive Drug	No.	Died	(%)	No.	Died	(%)	No.	Died	(%)
Vasopressor	26	22	(85)	78	68	(87)	17	10	(59)
Isoproterenol	1	1	(100)	7	7	(100)	7	5	(71)
Phenoxybenzamine	6	6	(100)	8	8	(100)	9	9	(100)
None	74	52	(70)	34	28	(82)	7	6	(86)

a large dose of steroid. An insufficient number of patients have been treated with vasodilators, such as isoproterenol and phenoxybenzamine. When used, these have been given after other agents had failed to cause improvement. Improved results can be anticipated with these agents, provided that serious complications are not present, the patient is treated early in the course of shock, and an appropriate antibiotic is selected.

Rationale for Steroid Therapy

The rationale for the use of pharmacologic doses of corticosteroid has not been clearly defined but the following points can be made: (1) The glucocorticoids have an anti-inflammatory effect, thus contributing to a reduction in fever and decrease in toxemia. The patients look and feel better. (2) Pharmacodynamic effects include a reduction in peripheral resistance, increased glomerular filtration rate, and an increase in cardiac output. The improvement in renal function with an increase in the output of urine can be dramatic. The effect of corticosteroid on the renal vasculature in canine endotoxin shock has been demonstrated by Sullivan and Cavanagh.[5] (3) Lysosome membranes are stabilized, preventing release of proteolytic enzymes and other deleterious factors into the blood stream. These enzymes may have a vasospastic effect and are injurious to other tissue cells.

Summary of Therapy

In summary, endotoxin shock must be recognized early in its course. Toward this goal, we are proceeding with the following regimen for management of endotoxin shock:

A. Measurements
1. Arterial pressure and pulse
2. Central venous pressure
3. Electrocardiogram
4. Urine output
5. Evaluation of renal function
6. Precise bacteriology

B. Treatment
1. Prompt administration of fluids; plasma and whole blood when indicated; usually physiologic saline
2. Appropriate antibiotic
3. Vasopressor drug—maintaining arterial pressure at 80–90 mm Hg systolic
4. Corticosteroid—minimum 50 mg/kg of body weight immediately, and then daily as a drip for 4 to 5 days
5. Digitalis—if venous pressure is elevated or if there is evidence of heart failure.

One of our most significant contributions to the management of patients with endotoxin shock at the University of Minnesota Medical Center is alerting the house officers and staff to the early recognition of shock. This factor, combined with appropriate therapy, has contributed to a gradual decrease in mortality.

REFERENCES

1. Spink, W. W., and Anderson, D.: Experimental Studies on the Significance of Endotoxin in the Pathogenesis of Brucellosis, *J. Clin. Invest.* **33**:540, 1954.

2. Thomas, L., and Good, R. A.: The Effect on the Shwartzman Reaction. I. The Production of Lesions Resembling the Dermal and Generalized Shwartzman Reaction by a Single Injection of Bacterial Toxin in Cortisone-Treated Rabbits, *J. Exper. Med.* **95**:409, 1952.

3. Spink, W. W., and Vick, J.: Evaluation of Plasma, Metaraminol, and Hydrocortisone in Experimental Endotoxin Shock, *Circulation Res.* **9**:184, 1961.

4. Weil, M. H., and Spink, W. W.: The Shock Syndrome Associated with Bacteremia Due to Gram-Negative Bacilli, *Arch. Intern. Med.* **101**:184, 1958.

5. Sullivan, T. J., III, and Cavanagh, D.: Corticosteroids in Endotoxin Shock, *Arch. Surg.* **92**:732, 1966.

Endotoxin Shock in Pregnancy and Abortion

DENIS CAVANAGH, M.D.

KRISHNA B. SINGH, M.D.

Endotoxin shock is usually seen by the obstetrician-gynecologist in association with septic abortion, chorioamnionitis, and pyelonephritis. These conditions are generally associated with a mixed infection, but there is agreement that the agent precipitating shock is usually a gram-negative organism such as *Escherichia coli* or *Aerobacter aerogenes*. The initiating factor in the pathogenic process is believed to be an endotoxin. Certainly, this lipopolysaccharide-protein complex will consistently produce shock in the laboratory animal, although the quality of the response tends to vary with the species.[1]

The pregnant patients, like the pregnant laboratory animals,[2] appear to be more susceptible to endotoxin shock, and some individuals are more susceptible than others. Some patients with coliform bacteremia show no evidence of shock, whereas others show the typical signs and symptoms even in the presence of repeatedly negative blood cultures. Thus, as in the case of the non-pregnant patient, the hemodynamic and other changes must be evaluated and the patient treated on an individual basis.

Although there now are numerous reports on the subject of

endotoxin shock, its occurrence in pregnant patients has been given scant attention since the original description by Studdiford and Douglas in 1956.[3] Indeed, only one large series has been reported.[4] In view of the paucity of information in this particular area, we would like to report our observations on 50 patients. In particular, the role of corticosteroids in the management of these patients will be considered.

MATERIALS AND METHODS

Fifty patients with endotoxin shock associated with pregnancy were seen over the period July 1, 1959, through December 31, 1967. The patients' ages ranged from 17 to 42 years, with a median age of 30 years. Their parity ranged from 0 to 13.

The criteria used for diagnosis were, first, demonstrable evidence of infection, and second, clinical evidence of shock with a systolic blood pressure of 80 mm Hg or less, and persistent for at least 30 minutes, with no other cause of shock being found.

Cases of transient hypotension were classified as mild and excluded from the study. Moderate shock was considered to be present when the systolic blood pressure was 50–80 mm Hg. Severe shock was diagnosed in the presence of shock symptoms and a systolic blood pressure of less than 50 mm Hg. About one third of our patients were in this latter group.

The pulse rates ranged from 60–170/min, with most patients maintaining a level of over 100/min.

In this series of 50 patients, the conditions leading to endotoxin shock were as follows: septic abortion (39), chorioamnionitis (7), and pyelonephritis (4). Septic abortion was found to be the most common cause of endotoxin shock. About 3% of our patients with septic abortion develop endotoxin shock.

The organisms isolated on blood cultures are shown in Table I. A positive blood culture was present in 54% of the patients although this is not considered to be essential for the diagnosis of septic shock.[5] In addition to blood cultures, urine or cervical cultures should be taken, according to the primary site of infection.

TABLE I. ENDOTOXIN SHOCK: ORGANISMS ISOLATED ON BLOOD CULTURES

Organisms	% Cases
Escherichia coli	35
Aerobacter	17
Proteus	15
Pseudomonas	10
Others	23

Gram-stained smears provide a useful guide to the preliminary choice of antibiotics and for the detection of *Clostridium welchii* infection.

CLINICAL FINDINGS

Now, what of the clinical manifestations in endotoxin shock associated with pregnancy? The symptoms vary even in the same patient, because the process is dynamic. Although a few patients progress rapidly to the terminal phase, three fairly distinct phases can usually be distinguished. These apparently correspond to the early and late phases of primary (potentially reversible) shock and to secondary (irreversible) shock.

Primary shock in the *early phase* is characterized by "warm hypotension." The patient is hypotensive, alert, and anxious. She is flushed and her temperature is usually in the range of 101–105° F. Not uncommonly, she sustains a rigor coinciding with a temperature peak. There is usually an associated tachycardia, but about 25% of our patients had a pulse rate under 72/min. Pulse pressure is satisfactory and the urinary output is good.

The *late phase* of primary shock is one of "cold hypotension." The patient is hypotensive, pale, and clammy. Her temperature often becomes subnormal. She gradually becomes less alert. Her pulse pressure decreases as the cardiac output falls. Development of oliguria is an indication of inadequate renal perfusion. Oliguria should always be regarded with alarm. In the present series, oliguria occurred in 11 of 50 patients (22%). The triad of hypotension, tachycardia, and oliguria is typically present in this phase.

Secondary shock occurs when the body defense mechanisms

fail or the therapeutic measures taken to combat the stasis in the microcirculation are inadequate, or both. The hypoxia damages the smooth muscle of the vessel walls and a secondary phase of dilatation occurs. This is followed by sequestration of fluid into the extravascular space in such quantities as to make it impossible to sustain an adequate circulating blood volume. This is the phase of *irreversible* shock. No amount of blood volume replacement will give adequate perfusion of the vital organs, and attempts to do so will usually precipitate acute pulmonary edema. Respiratory distress and coma are terminal features. As our diagnostic and therapeutic methods improve, obviously the number of "irreversible" cases will be reduced.

We have no special "Shock Unit," but the care of all patients with endotoxin shock is supervised by a "Shock Team." This ensures that all patients are seen by the same physicians and that the same general plan of observation and treatment is followed.

The procedures in patient surveillance are as follows:

1. The blood pressure is recorded and graphed on a bedside chart

2. The central venous pressure is monitored

3. A blood volume estimation is obtained

4. The urinary output is recorded hourly

5. Blood studies are done as indicated (serum electrolyte, arterial pH, blood lactic acid, and blood uric acid studies are useful).

TREATMENT

The patients described in this study were seen over a period of 8½ years. In that length of time there was standardization of the therapeutic approach, although changes in the method of management evolved with experience. The same general plan has been followed but it is modified to suit the needs of the individual patient. Our method of management includes the following:

1. Insure adequate oxygenation

2. Insure adequate fluid replacement

3. Metaraminol *or* isoproterenol given intravenously according to the needs of the patient

4. Glucocorticoids (dexamethasone 3 mg/kg/day *or* methylprednisolone sodium succinate 15 mg/kg/day) given to all patients

5. Digitalization carried out as necessary

6. When a removable septic focus is present, remove within 12 hours by (a) dilatation and curettage, or (b) hysterectomy, or (c) both procedures

7. Low molecular weight dextran, fibrinolysin, and heparin have been used in a few patients, but these measures still come under the heading of experimental treatment.

RESULTS

Surgery and General Therapy

In analyzing the results of treatment, the 50 patients were considered in two groups, and we concentrated on those patients who had developed shock as a complication of septic abortion. In this way we felt that we would be able to achieve a more meaningful detection of trends.

Group A, from July 1, 1959, through July 1, 1965, included 25 patients with endotoxin shock. Septic abortion was the cause in 18 patients, and of these, 3 died (17%). A dilatation and curettage procedure was performed in 15 patients, usually within 12 hours of admission. Two of the women ultimately required a hysterectomy and both survived (Table II). Medical treatment

TABLE II. ENDOTOXIN SHOCK: RESULTS WITH 18 SEPTIC ABORTIONS
GROUP A: 1959–1965*

Surgery	Survived	Died	Total
D & C	13	2	15
D & C and hysterectomy	2	0	2
None	0	1	1
Total:	15	3	18

* Over-all mortality 17%

consisted of giving intravenous fluids, antibiotics, corticosteroids and vasopressors. In view of the widespread condemnation of vasopressor drugs it is of some interest that the results appear to be better in pregnant patients. Metaraminol was used in 17 patients, with the mean dosage being 170 mg; 2 of these patients died. One patient who received metaraminol intermittently for 12 days survived; thus we are not particularly impressed with the hazards attendant on the use of this particular drug.

Group B, from July 1, 1965, through December 31, 1967, also included 25 patients with endotoxin shock. Of these cases, 21 were associated with septic abortion, including one death (4.8%). Dilatation and curettage was performed in 16 cases, and a hysterectomy was required in 5 cases (Table III). Intravenous

TABLE III. ENDOTOXIN SHOCK: RESULTS WITH 21 SEPTIC ABORTIONS
GROUP B: 1965–1967*

Surgery	Survived	Died	Total
D & C	16	0	16
D & C and hysterectomy	4	1	5
Total:	20	1	21

* Over-all mortality 4.8%

fluids, particularly 5% glucose in saline, were used. Blood volume studies were done earlier than in the Group A patients, and using these results and the central venous pressure readings, we began volume replacement early. Antibiotic dosage was considerably increased, with dosages of penicillin in the range of 10 million units, and 0.5 gm of chloramphenicol being given intravenously every 4 hours. All of the patients in Group B received dexamethasone 20 mg intravenously every 4 to 6 hours; this was discontinued abruptly after 48 to 72 hours in all but two patients. Metaraminol was used in all of these patients, but the mean dosage was less than 50 mg per patient.

The over-all results in 50 patients with endotoxin shock associated with pregnancy are summarized in Table IV. During the period 1959–65, five of 25 patients (20%) died, but during the

TABLE IV. ENDOTOXIN SHOCK: RESULTS IN 50 PATIENTS*

Group	Year	Survived	Died	Total
A	1959–65	20	5(20%)	25
B	1965–67	24	1(4%)	25
	Total:	44	6(12%)	50

* Over-all mortality 12%

period 1965–67, only one of 25 patients (4%) died. The over-all mortality in the 50 patients was 12%.

Glucocorticosteroid Therapy

It is with corticosteroid therapy that we are particularly concerned here. In 1964, Weil and coworkers[6] reported that high-dosage corticosteroid therapy reduced the mortality in endotoxin shock. Glucocorticoids appear to have the following five beneficial actions: they exert a positive inotropic effect; decrease peripheral resistance, increase tissue perfusion; increase venous return, and stabilize lysosomes, so preventing enzyme release, thereby reducing cell destruction.[7-11]

From this study of 43 patients with endotoxin shock treated with glucocorticoids, the following observations were made.

1. Choice of Steroid Drug and Method of Administration. Initially, hydrocortisone was used in a dosage of 1 gm/24 hr, and then was increased to 3 gm/24 hr. Later, synthetic steroids such as dexamethasone or methylprednisolone sodium succinate were used.

Some changes were made in the mode of administration of corticosteroids during the course of the study. At first, dexamethasone was given as a bolus of 20 mg intravenously every 6 hours. Later a 20-mg dose was given intravenously every 4 hours. As a result of animal experiments, it was then decided to give dexamethasone 20 mg intravenously, as a bolus, followed by a constant infusion of dexamethasone in a dosage of 3 mg/kg of body weight every 24 hours. We believe that improvement of renal perfusion is more sustained than when the steroid is given as a bolus every 4 hours.

2. Adverse Effects of Massive Glucocorticoid Therapy. In all,

43 patients with endotoxic shock were treated with corticosteroids. There was no evidence of delayed wound healing attributable to corticosteroids in any of the seven patients subjected to hysterectomy.

One patient showed some puffiness of the face after 72 hours, and one patient developed stomatitis after 96 hours. Both conditions cleared promptly following cessation of the drug.

One patient died of a massive hematemesis from acute gastric ulceration. Although this must be considered to be associated with steroid administration over a 10-day period, the presence of a nasogastric tube during this same period probably also played a part. In retrospect, it seems likely that if this patient had been more promptly treated by hysterectomy, neither the prolonged corticosteroid therapy nor the prolonged intubation would have been necessary.

In an effort to evaluate more adequately the effects of short-term massive glucocorticoid therapy, four patients treated with dexamethasone were studied for evidence of adrenal suppression. Following a priming dose of 20 mg intravenously, dexamethasone was given in 500 ml of normal saline to a dosage of 3 mg/kg body weight. The median period of treatment was 72 hours and the steroid was discontinued abruptly in all cases. Twenty-four-hour urine collections were made on the seventh day after corticosteroid therapy was begun. The 17-hydroxycorticosteroid levels averaged 6 mg/24 hr and the eosinophil counts averaged 323/cu mm. After the administration of 25 international units of ACTH in 500 ml of normal saline over an 8-hour period, the 17-hydroxycorticosteroids reached an average value of 20 mg/24 hr and eosinophils 73/cu mm. Thus, no significant adrenal suppression was apparent following high-dosage glucocorticoid therapy continued for a median period of 72 hours (Fig 1).

3. Effects on Survival. It is difficult to separate the effects of one drug from the combination of drugs used in the management of these patients. There can be little doubt, however, that coincident with the use of glucocorticoids there was an improvement in survival rate. It will be noted that over the period 1959–65, 3 of 7 patients who were not given steroids died, while only 2 of

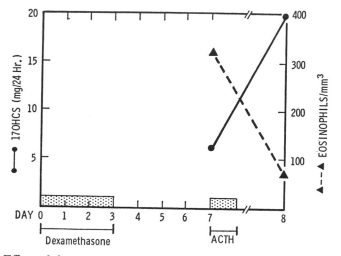

Fig 1. Effect of short-term (72 hours) dexamethasone treatment on adrenal function of patients with endotoxin shock.

18 patients treated with steroids died. Over the period 1965–67, all 25 patients received glucocorticoids, and only 1 died (Table V).

Laboratory studies on the renal vasculature of dogs and sub-human primates substantiate the belief that the kidney is a primary target organ in endotoxin shock.[12] Although it is not possible to say that glucocorticoids alone are responsible for the improvement in urinary output of patients with endotoxin shock, it is reasonable to say that they probably play a contributory role.

TABLE V. ENDOTOXIN SHOCK: RESULTS WITH GLUCOCORTICOIDS

Treatment	Group A (1959–65)	Group B (1965–67)	Total
No Steroids	3 of 7 died	—	3 of 7 died
Steroids	2 of 18 died	1 of 25 died	3 of 43 died
Total:	5 of 25 died	1 of 25 died	6 of 50 died

DISCUSSION AND CONCLUSIONS

The average mortality for septic shock of the endotoxin type is about 50%, the range being from 11% to 82%.[13, 14] The over-all mortality in this series of 50 patients was 12%, and for the last 25 patients it was only 4%. Our relatively good results in the management of endotoxin shock obviously cannot be attributed to better methods of observation or medical treatment, because essentially we follow the same plan of management as our medical and surgical colleagues. Most likely our success stems mainly from the following factors:

1. Our patients are young and have a firm grasp on life.

2. Although pregnancy appears to predispose to endotoxin shock, the condition may be more amenable to medical treatment in pregnant patients.

3. The patients are sometimes under our care when shock develops, and thus there is no delay in treatment as might occur during transfer to a "Shock Unit."

4. Our patients usually have a removable septic focus.

5. Pregnant patients with endotoxin shock may respond better to corticosteroids than nonpregnant patients.

From our experience in the management of these 50 patients with endotoxin shock in association with pregnancy, it is felt that, while it is important to follow a basic plan of management, the treatment should be tailored to fit the individual patient.

If a septic focus is present, it should be removed within 12 hours and the patient should be given antibiotics.

Glucocorticoids given in large doses for a median period of 72 hours produced no significant side-effects and appeared to be of definite value in the management of these patients. The principal manner in which these drugs exert their beneficial effect is unknown.

REFERENCES

1. Cavanagh, D., and Albores, E. A.: Intravascular Coagulation and Fibrinolysin Therapy in Endotoxin Shock, *Amer. J. Obstet. Gynec.* **92**: 856, 1965.

2. McKay, D. G., and Wong, T-C.: The Effects of Bacterial Endotoxin on the Placenta of the Rat, *Amer. J. Pathol.* **42**:357, 1963.

3. Studdiford, W. E., and Douglas, G. W.: Placental Bacteremia: A Significant Finding in Septic Abortion Accompanied by Vascular Collapse, *Amer. J. Obstet. Gynec.* **71**:842, 1956.

4. Douglas, G. W., and Beckman, E. M.: Clinical Management of Septic Abortion Complicated by Hypotension, *Amer. J. Obstet. Gynec.* **96**:633, 1966.

5. Weinstein, L., and Klainer, A. S.: Septic Shock: Pathogenesis and Treatment, *New Eng. J. Med.* **274**:950, 1966.

6. Weil, M. H., Shubin, H., and Biddle, M.: Shock Caused by Gram-Negative Microorganisms: Analysis of 169 Cases, *Ann. Intern. Med.* **60**: 384, 1964.

7. Lillehei, R. C., Longerbeam, J. K., Bloch, J. H., and Manax, W. G.: The Modern Treatment of Shock Based on Physiologic Principles, *Clin. Pharmacol. Therapeut.* **5**:63, 1964.

8. Robins, J.: Modern Concepts in the Management of Shock, *Obstet. Gynec.* **28**:130, 1966.

9. Spink, W.: Bacteremic Shock, *Hospital Med.* **2**:24, 1966.

10. Sullivan, T. J., and Cavanagh, D.: Corticosteroids in Endotoxin Shock, *Arch. Surg.* **92**:732, 1966.

11. Replogle, R. L., Gazzaniga, A. B., and Gross, R. E.: Use of Corticosteroids During Cardiopulmonary Bypass: Possible Lysosome Stabilization, *Circulation* (supplement) **33**:1–86, 1966.

12. Cavanagh, D., and Rao, P. S.: Endotoxin Shock in the Subhuman Primate. I. Hemodynamic and Biochemical Changes, *Arch. Surg.* **99**:107–112, 1969.

13. Coleman, B. D.: Septic Shock in Pregnancy, *Obstet. Gynec.* **24**:895, 1964.

14. Shubin, H., and Weil, M. H.: Bacterial Shock, *JAMA* **185**:850, 1963.

Clinical Experience
with Corticosteroids in Shock

Internal Medicine

Moderator: WESLEY W. SPINK, M.D.

Discussants: MAX H. WEIL, M.D.

JAMES C. MELBY, M.D.

ROLF M. GUNNAR, M.D.

JACOB FINE, M.D.

DR. SCHUMER

The first session of the workshop on Use of Corticosteroids in Clinical Management of Shock will be on internal medicine, with Dr. Wesley W. Spink moderating. The discussants will be Dr. Max Weil, Dr. James Melby, Dr. Rolf Gunnar, and Dr. Jacob Fine.

DR. SPINK

I see there are four internists to one surgeon—probably as it should be. This morning we had quite an interesting discussion; however, one man on this panel was not on the program this morning and I would like to introduce him. He is Dr. Rolf Gunnar, Professor of Medicine, and Chief of the University of Illinois Medical Division at Cook County Hospital.

This morning was provocative and productive, in both the basic and clinical material presented. Someone said to me this afternoon, "Certainly you would think there is nothing else but steroids for shock." My simple retort was, "That is why we are having this symposium; to discuss the steroids and their place in the management of shock." I think all of us agree that there probably is a place for corticosteroids in pharmacologic doses. We're not quite sure how they act. Many of us believe, from clinical observations, that they are effective. At this time, perhaps, I may ask whether there are any questions from the floor. If so, recite your name and ask your question, and we will call upon the appropriate individual to answer.

Measurement of Oxygen Consumption

DR. JULIA APTER, Associate Professor of Surgery, University of Illinois College of Medicine

I would like to know the feeling of this group about the need and efficacy of monitoring the oxygen consumption as an indication of either improvement or a tendency towards irreversibility in shock. I ask this because Dr. Fine's slides did not show that there was far more oxygen consumption in his subjects, and because this is one of the indicators for determining deterioration of the subject. On the other hand, Dr. Lillehei did not seem to be as aware of this oxygen consumption as an indication of degeneration of the patient, and some of his patients had an improvement in the oxygen consumption. Yet he instituted steroid treatment.

DR. WEIL

To start this discussion, I feel that blood flow and, in turn, oxygen consumption, is a critical issue.

DR. SPINK

If you can measure this at bedside, I'd like to know about it.

DR. WEIL

Dr. Spink's point is an important one. Before we concern ourselves with the measurement of oxygen consumption at bedside as an indication of the patient's physiologic status, we must find out whether we can determine oxygen consumption with sufficient competence to make this a worthwhile measurement.

If a patient had normal oxygen consumption, for example, 300 cc/min, and then exhibited a decrease in oxygen consumption of 5 cc/min, after 60 minutes he would have an oxygen deficit of 300 cc. This in itself might not be fatal, but by the time an oxygen deficit of 1,200–1,500 cc, or 2 liters, had occurred, there would be cause for grave concern. How accurately oxygen consumption can be measured thus becomes a matter of considerable practical importance. Even under reasonably refined clinical circumstances —as is well known to those of you who in older days measured the basal metabolic rate—a reproducible measurement of better than ± 10% cannot really be achieved. Under less refined clinical circumstances in the most critically ill, the direct measurement of oxygen consumption therefore does not really provide the needed accuracy.

An indirect measurement can be used. Cardiac output may be measured by one technique—such as the dye dilution method— and the arteriovenous oxygen difference may be separately measured by sampling blood from a pulmonary artery and a peripheral artery. This is equivalent to sampling in the pulmonary artery and in the pulmonary vein, and then calculating (by the Fick equation) the oxygen consumption that would occur at the given cardiac output; but even under those circumstances, we know that cardiac output measurements are only 15% to 20% accurate.

As if that were not enough, the human body, like any other machine, has an efficiency which is variable at different times; thus, oxygen consumption does not of itself indicate the oxygen need at a particular time. The patient may be under basal conditions or near-basal conditions at rest. Yet at one or another stage of the disease, he may be struggling, especially after problems of ventilation arise, as they so often do. The respiratory complications of shock probably cause more deaths on our ward than any other single complication. Even if an accurate measurement of oxygen consumption were available, it would not really tell us whether oxygen requirements are being met at a particular time.

For practical purposes, our group has concerned itself with the question of adequacy of the supply of oxygen to sustain aerobic metabolism. In the absence of adequate oxygen to maintain oxidative metabolism, lactic acid serves as the best available indicator of oxygen deficit.

DR. FINE

I was once interested in oxygen therapy, and although I have not concerned myself with it for a long time, I have a view on the subject. If the lungs are functioning properly, the arterial blood will be nearly fully oxygenated. But respiratory insufficiency is frequent. In that case one must assist the respiration by methods appropriate to the circumstances: for example, one may use a Bird or an Engstrom Respirator to prevent or alleviate atelectasis, alkali to correct acidosis, and tracheal aspiration to free the airway. Nevertheless, and in spite of such support, even including pure oxygen or hyperbaric oxygen, there will be a reduced oxygen supply to the tissues because the rate of peripheral flow is too slow. The oxygen difference between the arterial and venous blood rises to a varying extent, depending on where one samples the blood. Some venous bloods—for example, that in the hepatic vein—may show as little as 5 vol % and even less.

Effect of Corticoid on Clotting and Fibrinolysin

QUESTIONER

This is a question directed to Dr. Melby. What is the effect of cortisol on clotting and fibrinolysis?

DR. MELBY

I can't say what the acute effect of any of the steroids is on the clotting mechanism. There have been at least a dozen studies which have had completely opposite and equivocal results in terms of the clotting mechanism. We do know certain things about it. The fibrinolysin that is released may cause some changes in the peripheral circulatory physiology which are akin to those of endotoxin; and cortisol, when injected in pharmacologic doses into dogs, will completely reverse those changes. Actually, Dr. Spink and I did some of these studies earlier and didn't publish them; but there is a totally different problem associated with steroids that Dr. Takata perhaps mentioned: If the dose is reduced, some patients who have been on steroid therapy will show thromboembolic phenomena. This is a common experience; everyone who has given patients large doses of corticosteroids and then suddenly reduced the dose, has witnessed sometimes fatal thromboembolic phenomena. But this is unrelated to the acute effect, and I wonder if Dr. Cavanagh would address this question more specifically.

DR. CAVANAGH

I have been trying to find out something about this phenomenon for some time, and the only thing that I can offer is that reliable fibrinolysin activator is less common in the pregnant animal. It has been suggested that because the activator is less common, the profibrinolysin occurs in the clot in pregnant animals and disseminated intravascular coagulation cannot lyse the clot. Fibrinolysin problems are much less common in pregnant patients. When considering the part cortisone plays in the treatment of patients, one can only postulate that perhaps it keeps the lysosomes intact, and that the lysosomes are associated with proactivated substance, rather than fibrinolysin-activated substance.

DR. SPINK

Dr. Douglas, do you have any comments?

DR. DOUGLAS

We recently had the opportunity to study a few patients in endotoxic shock for the purpose of determining whether their blood was actually in the process of intravascular coagulation. Primary studies were those of circulating platelets, circulating fibrinogen, presence of free hemoglobin in plasma, the levels of plasminogen, and the evidence of active fibrinolysis in circulation. There was very conclusive evidence of intravascular coagulation, but in none of these patients was there an indication of generalized activation of the fibrinolytic system. Plasminogen levels were normal, as were the levels of plasmin inhibition. In contrast, however, in these pregnant patients, at least, there was very strong evidence of a localized activation of endotoxic tissues of the kidney.

Steroid as Vasodilator

DR. SPINK

Here is a question directed to me: "Do you use phenoxybenzamine hydrochloride for vasodilation, and what is the difference in the action of phenoxybenzamine and corticoids?" In the first place, I do not use phenoxybenzamine. Second, the preparation for intravenous use is not available on the market. It can be obtained as an investigational drug, so I would say under the circumstances, it has limited use. We have had very little use in this country. Dr. Lillehei, you did mention phenoxybenzamine this morning, and I understand that you are not using it any longer.

DR. LILLEHEI

I said I make great use of the steroids, and this is because they are easily available. However, phenoxybenzamine, an adrenergic-blocking agent, is very effective in decreasing resistance. It may also have inotropic effects, possibly due to driving potassium into the myocardial cells. There has been some work done on this. I think Dr. Spink has covered the reason why we do not use it. Perhaps it is not covered in a conference such as this because it has not been generally available. The other aspect is that with use of phenoxybenzamine, the degree of vasodilation can be determined, whereas steroids do not allow this measurement. I am not for a moment saying that with steroids their salutary effect is the result of vasodilation only. All I say is that in clinical use, steroids give a measure of one of the things they may be doing. If resistance is lowered with a massive dose of steroids, and a known alpha-adrenergic-blocking agent then given, and it is observed that the resistance does not change appreciably, there has been achieved a certain measure of vasodilation, as compared to this dose of phenoxybenzamine, which is usually about 1 ml/kg. So it is the initial action that I am trying to clarify, although the ultimate answer, I am sure, will be found at the cellular level, as Dr. Schumer, Dr. Fine, and many of the others have talked about. I might add that phentolamine will do the same thing as phenoxybenzamine, but it is even harder to use because it has to be given continuously, as the dose effect is over in a few minutes.

DR. SPINK

Would anyone like to comment on the use of phenoxyben-zamine?

DR. FINE

Dr. Lillehei has covered the use of phenoxybenzamine hydro-chloride very well.

I might add a note here about the futility of steroid therapy. So much depends on the state of the patient's residual resources for defense, especially for antibacterial defense, when the steroid is administered. This is a young field and we are only beginning to see the light. One should not expect to get anything yet from statistical analyses of data. It is quite clear that the steroids have their severe limitations. They will do remarkable things, but frequently they will not cure, because the lesion that they can correct is not the only one that needs correction. Thus in a patient with cirrhosis of the liver, antibacterial defenses are almost certainly depleted so that the steroids will not be useful. As I see it, steroid should be used to try to restore the structural integrity of the peripheral vessels. But from the data already in hand we can expect, despite restored integrity of these vessels, that relapse into shock will be frequent because of the additional injuries that the corticosteroids cannot repair.

The patient in advanced shock needs considerably more therapy than one in an earlier phase of shock. One must support the de-toxifying systems against further deterioration at least by block-ing bacterial activity, for example, by giving nonabsorbable antibiotics into the gut to reduce absorption from the gut and to relieve vasoconstriction of the liver and spleen as by extradural anesthesia or celiac block. But it may eventually prove necessary also to clear the blood of circulating endotoxin, either by implant-ing a donor spleen or by providing an equivalent substitute, such as a potent splenic extract, for the damaged reticuloendothelial system. Of course this kind of substitution therapy will be a long time gaining acceptance. Meanwhile, with accumulating experi-ence we should acquire a better perspective on the therapeutic potential of corticosteroid if used early enough and in a suffi-ciently large dose.

DR. SPINK

Dr. Gunnar, you haven't had an opportunity to say anything, and I wonder, since you are in a very important unit at Cook County Hospital, and see a wide range of cases of acute trauma, if you want to comment briefly on what you heard this morning?

Efficacy of Steroids

DR. GUNNAR

Thank you. I am a bit confused, and it concerns me that we are talking about two seemingly separate actions of steroids. We talk about their use as a vasodilator, and about another use which is an ill-defined action on the cell membrane: stabilizing lysosomes, improving oxygen consumption, and improving the contractility of smooth muscle. Up to this time, much of the work that has been done on the clinical use of steroids related to their action as a vasodilator. We have studied and are studying this problem. After physiologic doses of steroids were shown to have little effect in shock, we followed the advice of Dr. Lillehei and used at least the equivalent of 2 gm of hydrocortisone as a single injection for the vasodilator effect. We have studied 16 patients and found very little hemodynamic change. Now Dr. Lillehei tells us that 10 gm are to be used. But if the index used is vasodilation or decreased vasoconstriction, then there are other drugs which are equal or more effective, in our experience. Such drugs as chlorpromazine or phentolamine can be used intravenously, are available, and can accomplish the same purpose. If we are talking about the other actions of steroids as measured by survival statistics, there is good evidence in the experimental animal, using the endotoxin shock model over many, many years, that steroids are effective. Steroids are purported to be even more effective at higher doses, but in the human I do not see that there are as yet good survival statistics which will tell us whether that was the agent which really made the difference in survival. I am a little cautious in saying what steroids do, from the evidence that has been presented up to this point. I would like to go back to another statement that Dr. Spink made earlier. The real difference in studying these patients is that both intravascular pressures and cardiac outputs are measured, and it is possible from moment to moment to observe the effect of treatment on these patients. I think this is going to change survival statistics. One can see what the agent being used is actually doing hemodynamically, if hemodynamic changes are measured.

DR. SPINK

I assume that you do not use steroids in the treatment of shock at your institution.

DR. GUNNAR

We have, as I've said, studied 16 patients with 2-gm dosage. Seven of these were in gram-negative shock, five gram-positive, and one each myocardial infarction, pulmonary embolism, hypovolemia following circulatory arrest, and infection by undetermined organism (Table I). We found no evidence of any consistent change in hemodynamics with this amount of drug. We will continue to use steroids at physiologic dosage. I am anxious to find out what the direct cell-membrane effect is from investigators who are working at that level. But as a clinical investigator, I am not yet convinced that we should go to the dosage that has been suggested today.

DR. FINE

I think it is a mistake to try to take a position on steroids on the basis of statistics. This is a young field. The enthusiasm for steroids is just getting started because we're beginning to see a little light, and therefore this is a place where we ought to consider why one should expect to get nothing from statistics, at least in the beginning. It is quite clear that steroids have their limitations. They are not a panacea. They will do certain things, but they will not cure, because more than one lesion is being aimed at. The intention is to restore vascular integrity; but it is quite clear from the data that vascular integrity can easily relax if no account is taken of additional phenomena that are proceeding concurrently. Moreover, steroids will not work just anytime. With a patient who is well advanced in shock, it would be right not to use the steroid because it is not going to work in very advanced

TABLE I. HEMODYNAMIC MEASUREMENTS IN SHOCK PATIENTS FOLLOWING STEROID ADMINISTRATION

Patient	Age	Diag.	Dose/Time	Response to Steroid Therapy 16 patients						Control (Pre-Therapy)				
				%△ MAP	△CVP	%△ HR	%△ CO	%△ SV	%△ SVR	MAP	CVP	CI	SV	SVR
J.A.	60	MI	2 gm/30	−33	−4.5	−12	− 9	+ 5	−23	61	8.5	4.5	101	6.5
C.B.	45	g+	320 mg/90	+ 2	−3.5	0	+10	+10	− 2	64	12.0	5.6	77	5.5
P.B.	58	g−	200 mg/50	+13	−1.0	+ 2	+ 2	0	+10	60	8.0	3.8	59	10.0
W.B.	71	g−	2 gm/30	−24	+0.5	+ 6	+ 5	− 2	−28	92	5.0	4.5	125	10.2
P.C.	73	g−	400 mg/32	0	+0.5	− 5	−14	+ 3	0	62	4.5	4.3	98	7.8
R.D.	63	I	2 gm/25	− 7	−1.5	0	0	0	− 6	105	7.5	3.3	47	18.4
E.E.	68	PE	2 gm/30	+22	0.0	+ 5	+32	+28	−10	74	0.0	2.3	39	16.3
R.H.	53	g−	1 gm/70	−34	+0.6	−58	−67	−20	+82	94	9.0	5.8	122	7.3
W.H.	88	g−	2 gm/99	+40	+1.0	+16	− 2	−15	+45	72	8.5	6.6	98	5.1
F.J.	44	Hypo-V.	2 gm/28	−21	−1.0	0	+15	+15	−32	82	4.0	7.8	97	5.7
J.C.R.	57	g+	2 gm/60	+18	+1.0	0	+30	+30	−11	57	5.0	4.9	100	5.3
J.L.R.	42	g+	400 mg/26	+26	+2.5	− 3	− 7	− 4	+34	50	10.0	5.8	70	4.1
J.M.R.	69	g+	2 gm/64	0	0.0	+11	−17	−25	+16	60	3.0	5.8	92	6.9
D.S.	55	g+	2 gm/12	+45	+1.0	− 7	+89	+104	−23	40	2.0	3.1	51	8.1
L.S.	80	g−	2 gm/28	0	0.0	−10	− 7	+10	+ 7	59	0.0	1.0	10	42.0
H.U.	55	g−	2 gm/38	− 7	0.0	− 6	− 7	− 1	0	90	2.0	5.4	116	7.7
Mean	61		/45	+2.5	−0.3	− 4	+3.3	+ 8.6	+3.7	70	5.5	4.7	81	10.4
S.D.	12.5		/24	23	1.7	16	31	29	29	17	3.5	1.6	32	9.0

Dose shown in grams is hydrocortisone. Dose shown in milligrams is methylprednisolone.

MI—myocardial infarction; g+—gram-positive infection; g——gram-negative infection; Hypo-V.—hypovolemia following resuscitation for myocardial infarction; PE—pulmonary embolism; I—infection, organism undetermined.

Key to Column Headings: MAP—mean arterial pressure; CVP—central venous pressure; HR—heart rate; CO—cardiac output; CI—Cardiac Index; SV—stroke volume; SVR—systemic vascular resistance.

shock. The patient must still have some resources if a response is to be expected from the steroid. Once the response is gone, it might seem that this patient's condition is irreversible; but I take the position that even if the steroid fails, the condition is still not irreversible: there is still another lesion to treat, and that is the detoxifying or reticuloendothelial system. Failure of this system will probably kill most of these patients. So I would say if some kind of judgment is made as to what to expect from steroids, respect for their therapeutic potential might eventually be acquired.

DR. SPINK

We have been studying endotoxin shock for 15 years and, as I said in my remarks this morning, it is the hardest type of clinical investigation. Shock is dynamic. Many things are taking place. One must do certain things. I am convinced from observations that my colleagues and I have made that if one has a patient critically ill with shock—bacterial shock, endotoxic shock—and that if adequate fluid has been given, properly selected antibiotics, either vasopressor or vasodilator substances, and the patient does not improve, one is then committed to use large doses of corticosteroids. Although the basic information is lacking, we still have enough evidence at hand to indicate that the patient is benefited. As Dr. Fine said this morning, "It's the patient that counts." So, one thing we should take away from this symposium today is that a tremendous amount of work has been done experimentally and many clinical observations have been made, and it is not the type you can do with a double-blind study. I have enough trouble looking at one patient with two eyes. I think that in view of what has been done with steroids in shock, one is almost obliged to try these agents, knowing little or no harm will result. Now if anyone would disagree with my statement, that's fine. Dr. Fine, Dr. Lillehei, and I have attended past symposia that proceeded almost like revival meetings. They would all agree that shock should be treated, but there were different ways to go about it. The reason we don't know very much about definitive therapy is that we lack so much knowledge about the dynamic nature of shock.

DR. GUNNAR

I would like to restate my position so that I make myself clear. The point I'm trying to make is that if use of a vasodilating agent is indicated, a proven vasodilating agent should be used—if, on the basis of hemodynamic changes or other evidence, this is the action needed at the moment. I don't think we are going to find the answer to whether steroids are effective or not by looking at hemodynamic changes. It is perhaps evident to everyone now that steroids have a place in the treatment of bacteremic shock, and perhaps steroids should be given early to patients who are in shock, but I think it is not correct to use them as a vasodilator agent. I would prefer to see other vasodilator agents used. But when the steroids are used for their effects on intracellular changes or changes in cell metabolism, they should probably be given early, without regard to the hemodynamic status at that particular point.

DR. SPINK

Well, I almost succeeded in stirring up a controversy, but I guess there is agreement now. I think it is a mistake to call steroids vasodilators. We should be very clear about what we are talking about and should conclude that the biological effects of steroids in shock are poorly understood. Basically what we have learned here today is that the steroids probably act at the cell membrane level, including vessels, and probably have a role in the shift of fluids.

I would like to bring out a point that was raised this morning. Do we think that steroids have a definite place in the treatment of cardiogenic shock? I would like to ask the speakers or anyone in the audience if they know of any good evidence that the steroids are effective in myocardial damage due to coronary occlusion and infarction.

Are Steroids Indicated in Cardiogenic Shock?

DR. FINE

When we studied the vascular muscle by electron microscopy to see if we could identify a structural lesion, we included the myocardium. Guyton and his collaborators[1] have insisted that the heart is the site of the central lesion in shock, whether or not the shock is initially cardiogenic. If the heart is to be held primarily responsible, one should expect to find structural injury in the myocardium as we have been able to find it in the peripheral vessels, as a counterpart to the hemodynamic pathology. No structural change in the heart was apparent by electron-microscopic study. Improved cardiac performance after steroid therapy can be adequately explained as an indirect effect of improvement of the peripheral circulation.

The view that steroid improves flow because it is a vasodilator is not supported by experimental data. If steroid for any reason improves flow, vasoconstriction will give way and vasodilatation will follow. Objective measurements showing a good hemodynamic response are good clinical evidence of the effectiveness of steroid. But a cure of shock should not be expected from a good hemodynamic response alone.

DR. SPINK

The question was not about endotoxin shock and the effects on the heart muscle but rather the myocardial damage due to infarction and ischemia.

DR. FINE

That is low-output shock. Why should that be different, let's say, from the low-output shock from a pulmonary embolism?

DR. SPINK

In other words, you don't believe that the steroids have any effects in cardiogenic shock?

DR. FINE

Steroids should have a positive effect on damaged walls of the blood vessels in severe shock, no matter how the shock was caused. Even so, one cannot hope for much from steroid in shock due to acute myocardial infarction, since a heart lesion severe enough to cause shock is in itself likely to be fatal.

DR. GUNNAR

I would like to take exception here. I'm evidently going to be the devil's advocate. I think one of our problems is that we have tried to call all cardiogenic shock the same thing. Shock in myocardial infarction is one thing; cardiogenic shock following surgery, or the kind seen after a patient has been volume-repleted for hypovolemic shock—that seems to be another entity. Unlike the patients that have been studied by Dr. Lillehei, most of our patients do not have elevated peripheral vascular resistance when they are in shock associated with acute myocardial infarction. It is important for them to have normal or near-normal central aortic pressure because they have severe coronary artery disease. I think we are in trouble when we try to equate cardiogenic shock in animals, caused by producing myocardial damage, with what we see in the human being subsequent to infarction. We have given steroids to only one patient with acute myocardial infarction in shock. These cases are so unstable that it is hard to make any assessment of what steroids will do over a 30- or 40-minute period. We could not see that it made any difference in our patient.

DR. SPINK

There has been quite a lot of clinical work done along these lines, and my impression is that there is no real definitive evidence that anything reverses myocardial infarction in the human being with shock.

DR. SADOVE

I'm confused. I would like to see you all get together on what shock is. If Dr. Fine's statement is correct, that there is a common denominator here, then what is it? Is there an organ whose metabolic function is damaged? Isn't this the reason for the use of steroids?

DR. SPINK

Do you use steroids in patients with myocardial infarction and shock?

DR. SADOVE

We use it in every form of shock, yes.

DR. SPINK

What results have you had?

DR. SADOVE

Our results have not been statistically compiled at this time; however, if the investigations of many of our colleagues are valid, there is a protection of the cell against shock. This may be the result of increased perfusion due to the vascular effect of corticoids, or a true metabolic inductive effect. Since the common denominator of all forms of shock is a decreased perfusion to the cells of all organs, I see no reason why corticoids could not work in cardiogenic shock.

DR. SPINK

That is true. We agree with everything you have said; but the question is how much evidence do you have that in myocardial infarction with shock enduring for 24 hours, the corticosteroids benefit the patient? It isn't a question of whether they are desirable or whether we have a unitary concept of shock.

DR. SADOVE

Don't we have evidence that steroids are effective in shock, Dr. Spink? Don't we have evidence that there is a reversal, that there are changes in the mitochondria, that there are changes in cell membranes?

DR. SPINK

Well, we are really getting warmed up now!

Clarification of Role of Corticoid in Shock

DR. WEIL

I am very sympathetic with Dr. Sadove's viewpoint and I share his sense of discomfort. May I propose an analogy for purpose of clarification? If a patient who has aspirated a chunk of meat is admitted to the emergency room and he cannot breathe very well, the problem may be approached in one of several ways.

The physician may ask for a laryngoscope, visualize the tracheal obstruction and extract the piece of meat. Another physician may elect to do a tracheostomy. Another might suggest an oxygen mask to improve delivery of oxygen and reduce cyanosis. Indeed, the doctor may even strike the patient on the back to provoke a cough with the expectation that this will dislodge the aspirated food. I think we might look at the use of corticosteroids in a comparable manner. They may be indicated in the same direct way that laryngoscopy may resolve the problem of aspiration. On the other hand, they may be no more helpful, and may be even hazardous, in the way that an oxygen mask fails to resolve the problem of airway obstruction. Frankly, corticosteroids usually have a fourth or fifth place of relative importance for treatment of the patient in shock. I believe the same statement applies to all drugs used for the treatment of shock, with the exceptions of fluid and digitalis. If a patient is in shock because he has lost blood or fluid volume, he needs volume. If a patient is in shock as a result of severe congestive heart failure, he needs an agent that is effective in restoring myocardial contractility. To the best of our knowledge at the present time (as Dr. Spink pointed out), if a patient is in shock because he has an overwhelming bacterial infection, the task is first to control the infection and then to do the supplementary things which will sustain the patient until definitive improvement is realized.

In the treatment of shock complicating myocardial infarction, there seems to be little doubt that the chief problem is in the left ventricular myocardium, and that there is a deficit in the function of the pump. This leads to a sequence of peripheral vascular changes, part of which have to do with pooling of blood in the venous capacitance bed. The best way to manage this situation is to restore the contractility of the pump. It is necessary, however, not only to do that but also to mobilize the blood collected in the capacitance bed.

I should like to go on record that I do not recognize corticosteroids as a general panacea for shock, nor do I recognize any other single agent in this role. I favor their routine use only in the treatment of bacterial shock. In my opinion, an etiologic orientation, a search for the cause of shock, properly precedes medication. In the late stages of perfusion failure, which unfortunately are not often reversible with current techniques, corticosteroids are likely to have a place but, like the other weapons that we have, they are relatively weak. I am convinced, on the basis of our experience, that the immediate treatment of choice for shock complicating acute myocardial infarctions is not the use of corticosteroids.

REFERENCE

1. Guyton, A. C., and Crowell, J. W.: Dynamics of the Heart in Shock, *Fed. Proc.* (No. 2), pt. 3, **20**:51–60, 1961.

Obstetrics and Gynecology

Moderator: WILLIAM F. MENGERT, M.D.

Discussants: DENIS CAVANAGH, M.D.

CLARENCE D. DAVIS, M.D.

GORDON WATKINS DOUGLAS, M.D.

DR. MENGERT

I believe the obstetrician-gynecologist has a special interest in shock. In the first place, hemorrhagic shock is something we meet in the accidents of pregnancy and of labor, particularly when there is abruption of the uterus, which fortunately is not too common. We also meet the young woman who uses abortion for birth control. Obviously, statistics of illegal abortion are almost impossible to obtain, but it is estimated that there are between a half-million and one million illegal abortions annually in the United States. Probably 95 out of every 100 women who seek and find illegal abortion get by with no trouble, or with very little trouble; but an estimated 5% of them develop complications which force them into the hospital. This percentage means probably between 25,000 and 50,000 such admissions annually. In talking with Dr. Douglas a little earlier, I learned that the problem is increasing in New York City. Of these 25,000 to 50,000 who come to the hospital, probably 2% to 3% will die, many of them in endotoxic shock. A great many years ago, before there was much interest in shock, it was said that when an obstetric patient hemorrhaged, either pregnant or in labor, whether she lived or died depended

116

on what was done for her in the first ten minutes. In other words
—to repeat what has been emphasized all during this wonderful
day—shock demands promptness in diagnosis and promptness
in treatment.

Now, with that introduction, I would like to call on Dr. Davis to
tell us about the difference between shock from the viewpoint of
the surgeons and the internists and from that of the obstetricians.

DR. DAVIS

In 1936, we reported a 45% mortality in 20 cases of septic
shock, most of them obstetrical. Cavanagh reported about a
$33\frac{1}{3}$% mortality in 35 cases and Douglas, 22% in 50 cases. We
heard this morning that Dr. Cavanagh's experiences in more recent years are considerably better than that. Time does not permit
a detailed analysis of the difference in the type of cases we are
dealing with, but I would assume that the discrepancy in the data
is largely due to the severity of the cases. I would hope that this
is the case, since, as you can see, we came out far the worst. In
October 1966, Dr. Speroff and I summarized our management of
bacterial shock in septic abortion in *Connecticut Medicine* in a
matter of some three pages.

Following is a description of our general procedures in treatment of endotoxic shock.

General Procedures

Blood, urine, cervix, and wounds should be cultured when indicated. Gram smears are of utmost importance, because they
frequently give a good indication of the organism present, and
thus permit choice of a specific antibiotic. Other needed data are
complete blood cell count, urea nitrogen, electrolytes, fibrinogen,
prothrombin time, liver function tests, platelet count, clot formation and stability, and, obviously, blood type and crossmatch. Additional data are provided by a base line electrocardiogram, chest
and abdominal x-ray films to rule out a foreign body, gas formation, subdiaphragmatic air, and masses. Use of the Foley catheter
is of utmost importance in determining output. Delay in the in-
sertion of an indwelling catheter in the bladder may result in

failure to recognize anuria or oliguria. The specific gravity of hourly urine outputs should be charted, along with frequent recording of vital signs. A strict recording of intake and output is necessary because these patients can drown in their own fluids. Intravenous mannitol in a 10% solution is given if the urinary output falls below 30 cc/hr, and we think that physicians who do not like mannitol are physicians who give it too late. Our attitude, more or less, is that it should be given just before it is needed. A polyethylene catheter is threaded through the antecubital vein into the subclavian vein or superior vena cava for venous pressure. Continuous central venous pressure is then readily monitored, and should be kept in a range between 30 and 120 mm. Intravenous fluids are administered by using a three-way stopcock at the bottom of the manometer. Blood transfusion is not indicated except to replace blood loss. Plasma or plasma-expanders may be used to obtain a normal central venous pressure. If the central venous pressure is high with persistent hypotension, rapid digitalization is certainly indicated. Metabolic acidosis is best treated with intravenous sodium bicarbonate. It should be noted that respiratory alkalosis may mimic acidosis with compensatory hypoventilation.

Antibiotics. If the smear does not show what organisms we are dealing with, we then use a diverse antibiotic regimen:

Penicillin, 60 to 80 million units per 24 hours, given intravenously. One must consider the potassium content of these large doses, because there is 1½ mEq potassium per million units of penicillin.

Chloramphenicol, 3 to 6 gm/24 hr, administered intravenously.

Streptomycin, administered intramuscularly, 1 gm immediately, and 0.5 gm every 12 hours thereafter, unless there is oliguria.

Such massive doses of penicillin are usually effective against all gram-negative organisms except *Pseudomonas.* Reactions include central nervous system irritation and hyperkalemia. A sodium salt of penicillin is available and should be used whenever there is renal damage. Early chloramphenicol toxicity may be detected by the decreasing reticulocyte count.

Circulatory Management. We have had little or no experience with vasodilators so my remarks will be limited to vasopressors.

In view of the physiology of endotoxic shock, vasopressors may be undesirable since they produce excessive vasoconstriction with secondary ischemia. Nevertheless it is our experience, and the experience of several others, that survival rates have been improved with vasopressors. Metaraminol and levarterenol are agents of choice because of their inotropic action on the heart. These vasopressors are given intravenously in concentrated solution, the rate of administration being titrated against systolic blood pressure and an attempt made to maintain a pressure of 90 mm Hg. The use of phentolamine in conjunction with levarterenol is recommended to prevent local tissue injury.

Steroids. In many reports there seems to be a greater survival rate for patients receiving high doses of steroids. We have had no experience with the really massive doses that were spoken about this morning, although I daresay we will come somewhere near those levels in the near future. Our own version of massive doses would be 50 mg of hydrocortisone, or 2 to 3 mg of dexamethasone/kg body weight, for 24 hours by slow intravenous drip. Such doses apparently have an inotropic action resulting in increased cardiac output. Also there seems to be a vasodilation effect. We have had no instances of gastrointestinal ulcerations, although others have reported them. We have treated 12 of our 20 patients with steroids at the doses mentioned, and the mortality was essentially the same as for those who did not receive dexamethasone. These 12 patients, however, appeared to be considerably sicker than those who did not receive the dexamethasone. It is our clinical impression, then, that this is a beneficial procedure, particularly for the very ill patient.

At Yale, we have what we call a team approach to the treatment of endotoxic shock. As soon as this condition is recognized, the internists join us in the medical management of the patient. My main interest in endotoxic shock is a surgical approach. We use curettage as early as we dare; after 4 to 6 hours of antibiotic treatment, we curette the patient to avoid one of the conditions Dr. Cavanagh showed us this morning. We are now using a suction curette which, in our experience, cleans out the uterus considerably better than the conventional curette. We use a liberal amount of oxytocin: 1 to 10 ampules per liter of saline is not infrequent; sometimes we give more than 10 ampules. We use the suction curette when the uterus is relatively small (12-week pregnancy or less), and when there is a good circulating antibiotic level, and the patient's clinical condition is stable.

In our experience, the following indications for hysterectomy seem to be reliable: Attempted abortion with recent intrauterine injection of certain chemicals, that is, soap, detergents, turpentine, lysol, etc.; clinical deterioration following dilatation and curettage, unremitting high temperature, falling blood pressure, and oliguria, especially for the persistently tender uterus, or decrease in vaginal discharge. Usually within a matter of 12 hours, frequently less, it becomes obvious whether the patient is going to be helped by the D and C procedure, or whether a more radical procedure will be necessary. A tender uterus, especially with a closed cervix and evidence of intrauterine sepsis due to *Clostridium welchii*, usually demands more radical surgery.

DR. MENGERT

Dr. Cavanagh, Dr. Douglas, do either of you take any issue with this?

DR. DOUGLAS

No, not really.

Gynecologist's Approach to Shock

DR. MENGERT

Well, then, it's Dr. Cavanagh. You're the one who is going to tell us the difference between the clinical picture seen by the internist and the surgeon, and that seen by us, so go ahead and do that.

DR. CAVANAGH

One thing I failed to mention this morning is that 11 of our 50 patients developed oliguria. Of these 11 patients, 5 died. In other words, 5 of the 6 patients that we lost had oliguria. So I think it is extremely important to remember that as soon as a patient becomes oliguric, we should investigate the situation immediately.

We are now studying subhuman primates—baboons—and have found that when we inject endotoxin, the fall in blood pressure is not rapid, that is, not precipitous, as in the dog, but relatively slow. For the aortic pressure to fall 20 mm Hg took about 30 minutes in this particular animal. The central venous pressure changed little after the injection of a dose of endotoxin, 7 mg/kg of body weight.

The renal artery flow, which I believe is probably more important than the appearance of renal arteriograms, showed that when endotoxin was injected, there was a precipitous fall within about 3 minutes. This fell from 350 ml/min to about 10 ml/min, despite the fact that at the three-minute stage, there had been almost no fall in the aortic blood pressure. This suggests that, in the subhuman primate, and probably in the human, the kidney should receive a great deal of attention in endotoxin shock.

This morning, I talked about the importance of hysterectomy in patients with endotoxin shock, if the D and C procedure does not immediately improve the patient's condition. The reason that hysterectomy is sometimes required is because not infrequently the infectious process involves the uterine wall, and no amount of curettage is going to remove that septic focus.

A uterine biopsy specimen revealing gross evidence of septic thrombi in the veins of the myometrium indicates the need for hysterectomy. In the patients that we see, as distinct from those seen by the internist, the surgeon, or the urologist, a removable focus of infection is usually present, and in determining the prognosis this factor is extremely important. From our laboratory experiences with the baboon, and our clinical experiences, the target organs in the primate appear to be kidneys, liver and lungs.

I would like to say something about coagulation studies. The question was asked as to why some studies of animals in endotoxin shock show no coagulation changes. I believe the reason for this is that the endotoxin shock process is dynamic, and coagulation as well as hemodynamic factors fluctuate from one phase of the shock process to another. When we injected endotoxin into the baboon and then did the coagulation profile, we found that in 10 minutes there was a 50% decrease in the platelet count (from about

300,000 to about 150,000/cu ml). There was also evidence of a fibrinolytic process at 10 minutes. Yet, in the same animal at 4 hours, and quite definitely in irreversible shock, the platelet count was normal and there was no evidence of a fibrinolytic process. I think that this example highlights the difficulty we have when we make spot measurements in endotoxin shock, whether they be of hemodynamic or coagulation factors.

There are two other points I want to mention. One is with regard to the controversial discussion about the efficacy of vasodilators and vasopressors. Both vasodilator and vasopressor drugs probably have a place in the management of endotoxin shock, but at different points in the disease process. If the patient is in the warm hypotensive phase, she will benefit from vasopressors (mainly alpha-adrenergic). But if she is in the cold hypotensive phase, she will benefit from vasodilators (mainly beta-adrenergic) and blood volume replacement.

Another point that frequently arises is whether bacteriostatic antibiotics rather than bactericidal antibiotics should be used in a patient suffering from endotoxin shock. It seems logical that bactericidal antibiotics would be the wrong drugs to use since their use will presumably lead to the massive destruction of bacteria with the release of endotoxin in large quantities. In practice, however, it does not seem to make any difference.

One of the problems that obstetrician-gynecologists face is predetermining those few patients in whom endotoxin shock is likely to develop. For example, out of about 1,200 patients with septic abortions, approximately 40 will have septic shock. So we are talking about 3% or so of septic abortion patients. Thus, intensive observation of all patients with septic abortions, even those with temperatures of 102° F or higher, is not an efficient way of deciding which is the "high-risk" patient, because of the relatively low yield for the effort. Dr. Douglas described an epinephrine screening test but we have not found it as helpful as he has. If a reliable test could be developed that would spot high-risk patients, particularly those with a septic abortion, this would be a tremendous contribution to the management of this problem. I would like to hear Dr. Douglas comment on this test and any refinements of it that he may have developed recently.

DR. DOUGLAS

Treatment of this disease affords a very illuminating study of the patient *in extremis,* and one learns from each one of the cases. I would like to summarize a few thoughts on one aspect which bears on Dr. Cavanagh's question. It has been indicated by Dr. Spink and by several others that pregnancy may represent a special problem; I think we should discuss very briefly why this may be true, since these are cases that come to the attention of internists and surgeons, as well as obstetricians and gynecologists. There is, of course, the fact that these women suffering from induced abortion or from amniotic sac infections have been, until quite recently before their illness, young women in good health and therefore possessing good powers of homeostasis. This in turn raises the specific question—and I listened in vain this morning for the answer: What are the powers of homeostasis which permit one patient to respond to endotoxin in a very dramatic and sometimes lethal way, while others appear to tolerate it with much greater safety? We have asked ourselves this question, having had the same experience that Dr. Cavanagh has had. At Bellevue Hospital, 500 women come in every year with abortions. Some 60% of these patients are infected, and among these (due to infection with the same coliform gram-negative organisms that sometimes produce massive infections), an average of 2% to 3% of the patients will later have hypotension and shock. Study these as we will, we have not yet been able to find anything in their background which distinguishes them from the other 97%. There obviously is some very profound difference. But we do not know how to measure the homeostatic mechanisms, nor do we know how to test susceptibility.

Epinephrine Test in Diagnosis of Septic Shock

The test that Dr. Cavanagh referred to is one developed by Dr. Fritz Karl Beller and myself, in a search for some satisfactory means to identify the patient who is in endotoxin shock. These abortion patients come in with mixed infections, some from the gas bacillus as well as the gram-negative organism, and some in shock due to blood loss. We utilized an observation originally made by Dr. Lewis Thomas. If one raises an intracutaneous wheal of epinephrine in the skin of a rabbit and at the same time injects endotoxin intravenously, within 6 to 8 hours a massive hemorrhagic necrosis will develop at the site of the epinephrine injection. We adapted this finding by injecting 7 ml of fresh plasma from the infected patient into the ear vein of a rabbit, and raising the intracutaneous abdominal wheal of epinephrine. We found this to be a reliably positive test in clinical circumstances that suggest the patient is in endotoxin shock. But the interesting thing with these obstetrical patients—once the uterus had been removed, and the temperature and blood pressure had returned to normal—was that, according to the test, endotoxin could be detected in the circulating blood for four to five days after the hysterectomy. The astonishing import of this to me is the fact that these patients somehow lacked the ability to clear endotoxin from circulation. This macromolecule is one which ordinarily is excreted in the urine, or rapidly taken up in the reticuloendothelial system, and its persistence without a new source of elaboration for a week is highly surprising. As everyone knows, the reticuloendothelial system is very important in determining the manifestations of endotoxin in any patient, yet we have no idea how to measure the function of this system safely in the pregnant patient. We have no way of determining whether these patients with infected abortion have a depression of the reticuloendothelial system or not.

Finally, I would like to point out that in the obstetrical patient this complication does not usually develop outside the hospital. In our series, 70% came in with infected abortions and often with high fevers. But their hypotension developed within the first 12 hours after admission. It is this observation which leads me to suspect that there is something we are doing to these patients today which we did not do some 15 or 20 years ago. It may be the vigorous use of antibiotics, it may be the fact that we no longer are afraid to make an adequate pelvic examination in the severely infected patient. But something seems to be pushing these patients into endotoxic shock.

For the remainder of my comments, I will respond to a few questions this afternoon having to do with the relationship of this syndrome to the blood coagulation system and the fibrinolytic system. I think it is essential for this audience to keep in mind that to talk about endotoxin shock in the rabbit, the dog, or in the human being, is to talk about three very different things. For example, the fibrinolytic system in the rabbit does not compare at all with that in the dog or in the human being. Plasminogen, which is the precursor of the active fibrinolytic enzyme, plasmin, may be found in the rabbit at levels of about 80 Christiansen units. A figure of 8,000 in the human being would be accepted as normal, a hundredfold difference. If anything, the dog has a far more active fibrinolytic system than does the human being. Consequently, for study of intravascular coagulation the animal is chosen in which it can be displayed in its most impressive fashion; this, I think, is in the rabbit. There we have learned that the early presence of intravascular coagulation can be detected quite reliably by a series of determinations. If endotoxin is infused continuously, as Dr. Fritz Beller has done in our laboratories, one finds that the platelet count drops in a straight line right down to zero. It takes about 12 hours of continuous infusion to reach the zero point. In contrast, the fibrinogen level drops at first quite sharply; then at about 100 to 125 mg/100 cc it levels off, presumably being replenished from the liver. A far more sensitive indicator is the finding of free hemoglobin in the plasma. This we have discovered in our most recent cases, in small but detectable amounts, since a degree of hemolysis appears to accompany intravascular coagulation. But perhaps the most significant finding in these cases has been the relationship to urinary tract function: these patients become oliguric and the oliguria is by no means restricted to the period when the patient is in hypotension or shock. We have studied one case quite extensively: a patient who lost approximately 50% of her functioning nephrons in the course of intravascular coagulation, as documented by thrombocytopenia, hypofibrinogenemia, hemoglobin in the plasma, and a persistent rabbit test for endotoxin in the circulation for one week. Renal function studies ultimately confirmed that kidney function had been reduced by that amount.

In the continuing study of this problem and the effect of steroids (incidentally, I am going back and double my dose), we found that the major role of steroids is to support the patient long enough to permit us to proceed with the definitive treatment of the source of endotoxin shock. When infection occurs within the uterus, it is not simply on the surface of the interior of the uterus; when the placenta is infected, the membrane surface exposed to the circulation in that organ is enormous. That is why the patient with an intrauterine infection due to endotoxin is in great danger. Once shock develops, it can go very rapidly and it is urgent to take a definitive step to remove the source of the endotoxin. I believe that is perhaps the most important objective in treatment, and it is really the reason why Dr. Cavanagh has obtained such encouraging results in the last two years. He is treating these infections more aggressively than he did previously. Dr. Cavanagh, do you have any comments?

DR. CAVANAGH

Yes! I would like to comment on Dr. Douglas' tests and also on Dr. Spink's comment this morning about how human serum complements potentiated endotoxin. As I was telling Dr. Douglas, we used this epinephrine test and we did not find it useful in screening out the high-risk patients. But he reported a second finding in that paper, which may be a more important observation. He reported that human serum potentiated endotoxin in rabbits, and we found exactly the same thing. In fact, this potentiation was so unbelievable that we ran a good many more animal experiments than we had intended to, thinking there was some procedural error. We found that only one two-thousandth of the endotoxin dose was required for 50% of the animals to die if injected with endotoxin and serum, compared to injection with endotoxin and saline. So we needed only one two-thousandth part of the dose to get an LD50 when we mixed the endotoxin with human serum, showing definite potentiation of toxicity. I wonder if Dr. Spink might want to comment on that.

Immunology and Septic Shock

DR. SPINK

We have contended with this problem of why one patient with *Escherichia coli* in the bloodstream gets into trouble and another one just sails along with a little fever, perhaps, and maybe chills. And this is the partial answer to what you are saying. I think probably there is increasing evidence that this is an immunologic phenomenon and that some patients develop a hypersensitivity. There is no question with brucellosis: a patient or animal recovered from brucellosis, and given endotoxin intravenously, requires only very small amounts to develop hypersensitivity. This is clear-cut; it is similar to tuberculin shock in a patient, or to an animal with a positive tuberculin reaction. It takes very small amounts. So hypersensitivity is a factor.

We have seen two groups of paraplegic patients with bacteremia respond to treatment without going into shock at anywhere near the incidence of patients with other conditions. Despite the presence of indwelling catheters and the fact that the patients may have recurrent chills, fever, and bacteremia, it is unusual to see a paraplegic patient plunge into shock and die. We have not seen shock in 100 cases, and we are cooperating with the Veterans Service and others in trying to clarify these findings a little further, because they seem to indicate an immune mechanism. There is good evidence that hyperimmune serum will protect animals against endotoxin shock. Therefore, is it that they have repeated infection, repeated insult, so that they have developed a hyperimmunity which protects them?

Further, in evaluating our series of diabetics over a 10-year period, we had expected that they would be afflicted with endotoxin shock much more frequently than they actually are, although it is true that older patients may have endotoxin shock along with diabetes. Now, Dr. Cavanagh, I just do not know, but the evidence at hand would indicate that endotoxin shock does represent an immune mechanism. Not necessarily the orthodox type of antibody which induces a hypersensitivity, but certainly a complement is involved. And, it might be, in adding endotoxin to human serum by the activation of complement—and we think it is set free with the formation of what is known as antitoxin—that perhaps in the rabbit this is highly ineffective. We do not know, but think this is extremely important.

I would like to ask Dr. Douglas a question. In the literature there is a great deal of attention to disseminating intravascular coagulation occurring with bacteremia, especially with gram-negative organisms. Hence these patients go into shock. How does one make the diagnosis of intravascular coagulation on a disseminated basis and differentiate it from what we have been talking about? As far as I can find out from our own clinical material and from published reports, it would seem that purpura is an outstanding manifestation of intravascular coagulation: that is, bleeding has occurred. But the thing that perplexes me—and I have had no personal experience—is that clinicians writing on this say that heparin is the thing to use; not steroids by any means, but heparin. I cannot understand, if patients are bleeding, how heparin should affect them satisfactorily without doing something. Perhaps you might answer this for us, Dr. Douglas, because I believe it is very important.

DR. DOUGLAS

I will reply by summarizing a recent case. A patient entered University Hospital in New York in the 18th week of pregnancy, with a painless dilatation of the cervix. Her physician attempted to tie a suture around the cervix to close it, and in the process the membrane ruptured. The suture was removed, and the patient was given oxytocin for the next 48 hours. At this point, her temperature went up very sharply and her blood pressure began to fall. The patient was treated with steroids and her urinary output decreased sharply. The manifestations I have described, which are a decrease in platelets and in fibrinogen, and the appearance of free hemoglobin in the plasma, all were detected during this period. It was for that reason that we gave her 75 mg of heparin intravenously over a period of six hours. This is not a very large dose, but in the face of a thrombocytopenia and with the patient on the brink of a hemorrhagic diathesis, this was sufficient to push her clotting time completely out of sight. What urine was coming out turned into virtually gross blood and heparin was stopped immediately. I show this simply to indicate that the use of heparin is by no means an innocuous procedure to be undertaken in a patient who already has intravascular coagulation. If the use of heparin has value, it is probably in protecting the patient against this problem, rather than in treating it once it is in progress.

DR. MENGERT

I would like to raise one question. Everything today has been directed toward endotoxic shock. In hemorrhagic shock—and we do see it—where shock is from blood loss, whatever happened to intra-arterial transfusion?

DR. DAVIS

I guess we left that for you, Doctor.

Hemorrhagic Shock in Obstetrics and Gynecology

DR. MENGERT

Well, I am reminded of a patient who came to us with the placenta half in and half out. It was removed, and the bleeding stopped; 1,000 cc of blood were given intravenously. The patient's shock state continued. Then she was given an intra-arterial transfusion through the left brachial artery and after 25 to 50 cc of blood, her blood pressure picked right up.

DR. DAVIS

Isn't Dr. Collins of New Orleans the chief proponent for this technique in obstetrics-gynecology? He is the only one that I can remember who has written much about it.

DR. MENGERT

Well, I have seen it used a few times in hemorrhagic shock, not endotoxin shock, with dramatic improvement in the patient.

DR. LILLEHEI

It is the speed of transfusion. I think there have been many studies to indicate that if you force the same volume of blood in at the same time in the venous side as in the arterial side, there is not any really significant difference. The old theory was that you perfuse the coronaries, but I do not think there is one whit of evidence that an intra-arterial transfusion is any better than any intravenous given in the same volume and within the same reasonable period of time. I think the Russians still write on it occasionally but there is no real basis for its use.

Fetus and Endotoxic Shock

DR. MENGERT

We have a question here from a medical student; it is a multiple question. "What effect on the fetus is seen as internal septic shock begins and progresses to completion? Does endotoxin pass the placental barrier?" Another: "What specific effects, if any, does it have on the placenta?" Another: "Is premature birth indicated to preserve the fetus or the patient with internal sepsis?"

DR. DOUGLAS

I will be glad to try to answer these questions. As for the effects of endotoxin shock on the living fetus, one very seldom has the opportunity to study this, because such cases are either abortions or sac infections, generally accompanied by the rapid demise of the fetus, either through direct damage or through the mechanism of the febrile illness. Occasionally, however, one does see such a case. We had one in Bellevue last year. A woman in profound hypotension, with pressures in the range of 60/40, with a urinary tract infection, was given high doses of steroids as recommended today, and simply observed. She had a gradual recovery and carried the baby for another six weeks, when it was born normally and in good condition. That shows that under some circumstances, apparently, a pregnancy can survive this cataclysmic event. In animals, at least, endotoxin affects the placenta very severely, increasing its permeability to the extent that quite large particles can pass; a colloidal carbon, for example, will go across a placenta perfused with endotoxin. I believe that the question of whether premature delivery is indicated to preserve the fetus in the face of maternal sepsis has so many qualifying aspects that it would be not very useful to discuss it, except to say that the intrauterine fetus does not tolerate maternal sepsis of profound degree for very long. Consequently, if the fetus is at term and one has the opportunity to induce an early delivery, one should certainly do so. There is a particular complication in the use of high doses of oxytocin, as Dr. Clarence Davis mentioned. Occasionally, when infection has penetrated into the myometrium, the contractions stimulated by oxytocin will deliver a bolus of endotoxin into the circulation and such patients have been known to go into deep shock almost within seconds of the start of infusion. This danger must be kept in mind.

Low Molecular Dextran in Shock

DR. MENGERT

Another question addressed to you. "Do you have any information on the use of low molecular weight dextran in disseminated intravascular clotting?"

DR. DOUGLAS

I do not. Do you, Dr. Cavanagh?

DR. CAVANAGH

No, I do not. I believe, however, that low molecular weight dextran is generally felt to be useful. I think that it does reduce sludging and gives a temporary replacement of blood volume which might be very useful in a patient who is hypovolemic with endotoxin shock. Dr. Davis?

DR. DAVIS

I have had no experience.

DR. MENGERT

Any more questions from the floor?

QUESTIONER

How about dextran? Is it contraindicated in pregnancy?

DR. CAVANAGH

No, it is not. I would like to comment on that earlier question about premature delivery. I think it certainly would be indicated, especially in a patient with chorioamnionitis. It would be essential to remove the baby in order to remove the infected placenta and membranes, and if necessary even the uterus. In a patient with pyelonephritis near term, delivery of the baby is definitely indicated to take the pressure off the ureters and let the renal pelves drain. I think that premature delivery is definitely indicated under both sets of circumstances.

I might point out just one thing. The fetus tolerates shocklike blood pressures fairly well if they do not come in too short a period of time. The fetus has been lost by several patients after automobile accidents in which they lost large amounts of blood. We had one very interesting observation. A pregnant patient being operated on for a berry aneurysm, under hypothermia, was cooled off in a matter of 3 to 4 hours; the operation took about 3 hours and she was warmed up again. We had fetal electrocardiograms going along with maternal electrocardiograms, and the fetal heart rate slowed on a 2 to 1 ratio right down until the maternal pulse rate was around 80 and the fetal pulse was around 40 for several hours. This baby was born two months later and was perfectly normal. So, if the pulse goes down slowly, the fetus tolerates it well. If it goes down rapidly—well, that is another thing.

Surgery

Moderator: WILLIAM SCHUMER, M.D.

Discussants: WILLIAM C. SHOEMAKER, M.D.

RICHARD C. LILLEHEI, M.D., Ph.D.

WILLIAM DRUCKER, M.D.

DR. SCHUMER

This is our final workshop. For this session we have Dr. William Shoemaker, Professor of Surgery at the University of Illinois College of Medicine, and again, Drs. Lillehei and Drucker. I will be the moderator.

Dr. Lillehei, would you like to discuss the use of corticoids in myocardial infarction shock?

Corticoids in Myocardial Infarction Shock

DR. LILLEHEI

Perhaps I should start with myocardial infarction. The statement was made in the Medicine panel that myocardial infarction really is not at present an indication that steroids should be used, and I believe that is probably a conservative, and certainly a not unjustified, opinion. However, I have served on a number of these panels in my years of studying shock and have heard these same statements made repeatedly for different types of shock. The main objection was that the original hemorrhagic shock models of Wiggers and Fine were modified when many of us used them; however, everybody modifies something slightly when they take it over.

DR. SHOEMAKER

Speak for yourself, Dr. Lillehei.

DR. LILLEHEI

The objection was that these models just were not any good. Man was different. We soon found, however, that man reflected pretty well what was found in the animal. There was no real distinction between the reactions of animals and of man to blood loss and fluid loss. So, that settled that. Then the next argument, some years ago, was that endotoxin shock in the animal was a completely artificial system and did not actually reflect what happened in man, and that there was no real reason to proceed with new programs for treating septic shock, despite the fact that the mortality was practically 60% to 100%, depending on how one defines it—let us say 60% conservatively—and this attitude has not changed in roughly 30 to 40 years, antibiotics or no antibiotics. When the data began to accumulate, it was found that man really was not so different from the animal. There were some exceptions to the general hemodynamic pattern that we would see in the dog, particularly the low resistance and high output, probably due to shunting. I think shunting also occurs in the lung in almost any human who has had sepsis, or it can occur in the peritoneum or in the pelvis with septic abortions or peritoneal swelling, from whatever cause. The same general findings in hemodynamics found in the animal also appeared in man, and we found that the programs that tended to work in animals tended also to improve human survival. I say tended, because we do not have enough patients yet to say definitely that in septic shock steroids are the thing, or a statement of that nature. We have indications, as Dr. Spink has shown, toward this trend in 1,000 patients studied.

From there, then, the argument became: "Well, maybe endotoxin shock in man and in the animal is not quite so different as we thought, but there is a real difference between cardiogenic shock in man and in animals. Now, here there is a real difference." I think the pattern is evident; that there is repeatedly an objection to the model. Granted, there should be, but once a reasonably good model is worked out, I think the next step is to apply it to the patient, especially if the condition is one of cardiogenic shock, which has a poor prognosis. It would be different if we were dealing with 10% mortality from myocardial infarction in shock, or 10% mortality from cardiogenic shock occurring after bypass surgery as such. But we are dealing with a mortality of 60% to 80%. We have a firm foundation in the laboratory and we have worked on myocardial infarction for several years. There is no doubt, I believe, that steroids increase survival in myocardial infarction and shock in the laboratory; and there is an indication that this holds true in man. What we need are more patients, but more experience will be in the same direction.

The increase in survival rate would appear to result not necessarily from a basic effect on the heart, but from something that makes the heart work a little easier, reducing cardiac work and reducing resistance. "The heart is a pump, not a music box," Lord Russell Bing said many years ago, and it has been hard to convince some that this is true. If we reduce the workload of the pump, it is going to last longer.

I know we need to study more patients in myocardial infarction. We are quite certain that this salutary effect of steroids occurs with cardiogenic shock after surgery, and I do not think it is in any basic way different from myocardial infarction in shock. We need the patients and we hope that within two or three years a planned study in one large St. Paul–Minneapolis hospital that sees most of the patients who have infarctions, or a large share of them, will give an answer on an alternate basis. As far as Dr. Shoemaker's study is concerned, there is no one that has better data than he; but I believe the models are a little different—for example, he always tries cortisone last, after everything else has been tried. I do not know if this makes any difference: that is one of the many things that studies with greater numbers of patients will answer. We do know that if a patient is not treated early, his chances of responding are less. As a matter of fact, we think we can resuscitate almost every patient, at least temporarily. The question is, is the basic problem correctable? The volume can be restored, but can the infection be cleared? Has a wrong-sized valve been put in? Is the infarction so large that there is not enough pumping area left? We know this is not true in most infarctions. The size of the infarction is usually correlated with the clinical findings.

Are Corticoids Effective?

DR. SHOEMAKER

We do not have a natural prejudice against cortisone. It is simply a natural caution and a modest belief that scientific principles should be applied before rushing to conclusions, as frequently occurs with clinical enthusiasts. We have given hydrocortisone as the first therapeutic agent as well as the last. As a matter of fact, we try to randomize the order of the therapy. Moreover, we have attempted to analyze the interactions of hydrocortisone with other agents. For example, we would like to know if it potentiates the sympathomimetic agents. We have attempted in a systematic way to evaluate the possible interaction by observing the response to the sympathomimetic agents before and after hydrocortisone, but have not found clear-cut evidence of a potentiating action of this drug.

This is an entirely different position from reporting the apparent good effects of hydrocortisone in patients that have been given many other drugs and fluids at the same time, "polypharmacy style"; everybody decries this approach, yet it is frequently employed. There is no objection to making "grade C" clinical observations; for example, after hydrocortisone administration the patient appears to be better. Nothing is wrong with this observation, as an observation, if this is all the information that is available. But until more objective evidence is forthcoming, we must remain unsatisfied as to the action of the drug, and its precise indications and contraindications. When some of these questions can be answered, we will have a more rational approach to steroid therapy. At this time we do not believe that it has a major hemodynamic action in the average clinical shock and trauma patient. It may well have a metabolic action. It may tend to correct acidosis by increasing hepatic glucose output, and increasing rates of lactate and pyruvate clearance by the liver. There may be many other possible actions far more subtle than we can gather from the presently available studies. Other than the occasional isolated patient, who may have been on the way to improvement without steroid therapy, I see no statistically significant hemodynamic effect of the agent given in either ordinary or massive, so-called pharmacologic doses. Moreover, I still view with great skepticism the attempts at giving large doses of steroids indiscriminately, and to every shock patient, and then when the patient looks a little better the next day, to say this is a great success for steroids.

I would like to make one other comment with regard to a previous speaker's comment on the possibility that there may be peripheral arteriovenous shunting. We are all intrigued by the possibility of shunting, which at present remains an interesting, but unproved, theory. There are a few specific conditions in which arteriovenous shunting is known to occur; for example, from the hepatic artery to the portal vein in hepatic cirrhosis, and arteriovenous fistulae following direct injury to large vessels. As yet, there is no direct evidence of peripheral A-V shunting in clinical shock, with the possible exception of the microcirculatory studies on the scleral conjunctiva. There may well be shunting in some types of shock but we have no basis upon which to conclude that it does occur. The shunting that was mentioned—that is, across the lung—is a physiologic shunting in the sense that the blood is not oxygenated, rather than being an anatomical A-V shunt. It really should be called pulmonary venous admixture, in order not to confuse this with anatomical A-V shunting.

DR. SCHUMER

I would like to take the prerogative of moderator and state that the biochemical effects of cortisone are more profound than you have implied. Some of the microcirculation studies we have done in humans and in rats are highly significant. Microcirculation is the common denominator in shock. Dr. Drucker, I wonder if you could comment on the effects of cortisone on renal function, which you mentioned in your discussion.

DR. DRUCKER

This is a subject that we can spend weeks discussing, but I think everyone recognizes that the kidney is organized as a wonderfully complex system to preserve circulating fluid volume, and the general mechanisms involved are known to second-year medical students. But they are not known completely by anyone; hence this is still a fertile field for investigation. Cortisone acts—it is not the primary action of cortisone—as a mineralocorticoid. But John Leutcher said that another hormone must exist to account for the adrenocortical effect on the kidney. In time, aldosterone was discovered. The mechanism for release of aldosterone is via a very sensitive device in the kidney, the juxtaglomerular apparatus, a baroreceptor system, very similar to the baroreceptors in the carotid vessels and in the heart. These receptors detect changes in arterial pressure. In the kidneys, the activity of the baroreceptor controls the liberation of a hormone which, in turn, controls the adrenal release of aldosterone; the net result of aldosterone release is renal retention of sodium and, consequently, of water. There is some question, when large doses of glucocorticoids are administered at the level advocated for the treatment of septic shock, whether at these dosage levels there is a detrimental effect upon salt retention. If it is kept in mind that Dr. Spink advises giving a large dose for a short period of time, there should not be any real problems with renal retention of salt in that relatively short period of time. There might be a question whether retention of salt and water is so undesirable, in view of the discussion today, in which some enthusiasm was expressed for expanding plasma volume in the treatment of septic shock.

Corticoid Effect on Renal Function

DR. SCHUMER

Beautifully put, Dr. Drucker. Now Dr. Lillehei, one of the problems that we faced in our studies was the occurrence of stress ulcers and of bleeding despite the fact that we did not give the "one bolus" steroid therapy. As a matter of fact, we gave only 2 mg/kg to our patients, but 6 of 50 patients developed stress ulcerations. I worked in a county hospital and I am now in a VA hospital, and we have to consider the nature of the population, but I know that you did not have half this much difficulty with your patients. Would you comment on it?

Complications of Corticoid Therapy

DR. LILLEHEI

I do not know what the answer is, because we have not noticed any significant increase in stress ulcers, or bleeding from other areas in the gastrointestinal tract, or in healing with this type of therapy. In any group of patients in shock, there probably might be about 3% or 4% suffering gastrointestinal complications. Maybe that is low or maybe that is high. But we have not seen any relationship. Why do you see it? Do you have a different type of patient? I do not believe, however, that, where you are dealing with a mortality of 68%, even if we accepted what you found, it would be a deterrent to the use of corticoids. I think it would still be justified.

There was one other point I wanted to make when we were talking about septic abortion. There is a definite need for early renal dialysis when the patient is being resuscitated. We have had three young women in septic abortion who were resuscitated, apparently with steroids, and had restoration of good skin color, good cardiac output, warm, pink, and changed from being obtunded to clear-thinking, but oliguric. We immediately effected renal dialysis. Our latest patient, an 18-year-old girl, was dialyzed within 5 hours after being admitted to the hospital. We got her out of shock. We noted that there was a continued oliguria; actually, an anuria. Arteriovenous shunts were put in, in the evening, and she was dialyzed. One does not necessarily have to hemodialyze for that. One can peritoneally dialyze. The important thing is early dialysis, particularly in a septic abortion patient, who can usually be resuscitated. But if the patient dies, as was mentioned by the previous speakers, it is the result of renal failure. This is true with older patients, too. Sometimes, during resuscitation efforts they get more fluids than the kidneys can eliminate and they will have to be dialyzed as well.

DR. SCHUMER

Dr. Shoemaker, I know you have done metabolic studies on these patients. Do you differ with any of the data presented this morning on the metabolic effect of corticoids?

DR. SHOEMAKER

I think the subject and the presenter should be commended. It was very excellent work.

DR. SCHUMER

Thank you.

DR. SHOEMAKER

I have very little to comment on. I think most of the work was done on tissue slices from experimental animals. Obviously, the important problem is to get some insight as to how this information bears on the energy state in the critically ill patient, and to what extent this may be effected either by the natural outpouring of endogenous hydrocortisone or administration of exogenous steroids.

DR. SCHUMER

Doctor, do you have a question?

Antibiotic Therapy

QUESTIONER

Yes. Suppose a patient, 30 minutes after cystoscopy, goes into shock and develops a fever as high as 105° F. What antibiotic therapy would be indicated?

DR. LILLEHEI

I think not necessarily antibiotic therapy, but certainly fluids. That was outlined fairly well by the speakers this morning. It depends on the bacterial flora involved, but *Klebsiella, Aerobacter,* and *Pseudomonas* are common; or *Pseudomonas* may be responsible, if a patient has a urinary tract problem. In such a case polymixin and kanamycin therapy should be started immediately. We have given kanamycin intravenously, switching to intramuscularly as soon as the patient is out of shock. I have not seen any problems. Dr. Spink, is giving kanamycin intravenously an unnecessary risk?

DR. SPINK

No, we use kanamycin intravenously. We are very cautious. It should be used when dealing with *E. coli* and the *Klebsiella-Enterobacter-Serratia* group. Kanamycin appeared to be effective in our series. We have used it intramuscularly and subcutaneously, but for shock we give 3 to 6 gm in a slow intravenous drip. After all, we are trying to save a life, but we appreciate the potential renal toxicity.

DR. SHOEMAKER

Dr. Spink, do you wait until you get the culture and sensitivity results before you start this therapy?

DR. SPINK

The most important approach in patients who do spike a temperature of 105° F with chills and fever after cystoscopy is to get a urine specimen first and with the gram stain examine it microscopically. The most commonly encountered organism is *E. coli*. We prefer to start with tetracycline, because most strains of *E. coli* are sensitive to this antibiotic. Kanamycin is also useful, and is used intramuscularly if the patient is not in shock.

QUESTIONER

Yes, he is in shock.

DR. SPINK

Well, then we give it intravenously. Another point that we should not forget is that these patients at times develop staphylococcal bacteremia. Many patients die eventually of a hospital strain of *Staphylococcus* that is highly resistant to antibiotics. So we also use one of the synthetic penicillins. Therefore, we use tetracycline, kanamycin, and penicillin. Penicillin will take care of about one-half of *Proteus* organisms and tetracycline the other half, so the combination of penicillin and tetracycline for *Proteus* is indicated. For the *Klebsiella* group we give kanamycin, and for *E. coli,* tetracycline. Does that answer your question?

QUESTIONER

What is your dose of penicillin?

DR. SPINK

I usually give up to 10 million units intravenously.

DR. DRUCKER

I suspect that much of the confusion that we have had here arises from the fact that we are dealing with some very complex clinical situations, and in the excitement caused by a desperately ill patient we sometimes overlook the rather fundamental precepts of treating infectious diseases which we learned in the early days of antibiotic therapy. I am really disturbed with the low rate of positive cultures in patients with septic shock. I think it was only 50% in Dr. Spink's series, and he is one of the country's foremost clinical bacteriologists. I think we might do better than that. One blood culture a day is a relative waste of time under these circumstances, if we are seriously interested in obtaining a bacteriologic diagnosis. Several blood cultures in a series—five or six a day— are the minimum needed. There is not always a relationship between the degree of fever and the reward of a positive culture. If we are worried about the urine, as is frequently the case, it is essential that urine be obtained fresh, spun down, and stained with both the gram stain and methylene blue. Why both stains? Sometimes, organisms are so damaged that they will not take a gram stain, and yet they still have morphologic characteristics which can provide useful information. When the urine is cultured, all too frequently a residual level of antibiotic in the urine inhibits growth on culture media. Also, if we stain the urine, we may learn that bacteria are present long before the cultures are mature. Another reason for frequent blood cultures with a patient in septic shock is that one does not have time to await the results of a leisurely routine; not one culture a day, but, ideally, seven or eight in one day.

Vasopressors vs. Vasoconstrictors

QUESTIONER

In endotoxic shock there is a concept that maintains: "First of all start with intravenous fluids and the appropriate antibiotic, then either vasopressors or vasodilators." How do you make up your mind whether to use a vasopressor or vasodilator?

DR. DRUCKER

I think everyone will agree that if the patient is constricted and cold, vasopressors should not be used.

DR. SHOEMAKER

I would like to answer that question. I think it is extremely difficult to find out whether the patient is constricted or dilated, on the basis of clinical observations. I think more precise measurements of the total peripheral resistance and cardiac output will elucidate more satisfactorily what state the patient is in. There are a few instances in which a patient has a low output with a high resistance and at the same time has hypovolemia. If this syndrome is associated with hypovolemia, then there is no substitute for blood volume replacement. But under no circumstances should a patient with hypovolemia be blocked. Some of our more advanced cases of shock were referred to us from another department after having been so blocked. Less than 10% to 15% of the patients in our series have this type of shock. More commonly the shock patients of our series have high outputs with very low resistance.

I think that phenoxybenzamine is a more effective blocker, but it lasts 18 hours or more. Some of the short-acting, milder blockers such as phentolamine or chlorpromazine may be used to evaluate the patient's hemodynamic status. But I do not believe that these patients should be blocked without having their cardiac output and resistance monitored.

DR. LILLEHEI

The cardiac index is worthwhile for indicating peripheral resistance because, I believe, it is the only way clinicians can be convinced that something has happened. The deterioration or the improvement attributed to various drugs can be observed. But we have to remember exactly what we are measuring. For example, total peripheral resistance is a derived figure. It is not a specific direct measurement, but rather, a formula derived from the pressure in the artery minus the pressure in the vein, divided by the cardiac output, times a constant; this can be a very specious figure, as we see in septic shock. With very low resistance, the patient can be oliguric, anuric, cold, clammy, obviously having very poor visceral and cutaneous circulation. Peripheral resistance may be around 500, and yet there is poor flow—and I think this is where I differ again with Dr. Shoemaker. The clinical impression is as valuable as the exact figure. In other words, it would be just as bad to treat these patients from the derived numerical data as not to have any numbers at all. We need both; but if treatment is deferred until cardiac output can be measured, and then total peripheral resistance calculated—then there will be a long wait. Most hospitals do not have this equipment, and there is not available the free labor—that most of us have in university hospitals—to do these things and stay up all night to do them. I do not think we should delay treatment to obtain such figures. On the other hand, this does not mean observations should not be made at the bedside. As for the significance of this resistance, again I think it is a specious figure, particularly in septic shock. We do not know what it means; it is the sum of resistance in the kidney and the lung and if there is shunting—arteriovenous shunting, of course—there will be high flow but no perfusion of tissues.

Now the question of when to use steroids. I do not believe anybody can say. Everyone has to make up his own mind about how to use this sort of therapy. I do not want to leave the impression that I believe that, because steroids are indicated in shock, they are the only drug therapy. I do think they happen to be the most convenient drug that we have to treat the patient in shock who does not respond to fluids. Now there are probably better steroids; there will, I hope, be other drugs, which will have the same or better effects, and I hope we will know exactly how they produce their effect. But at this moment I think the steroids are the most useful drug available to us.

The treatment of shock still depends on maintaining pressure by a good relationship between flow and resistance. Pressure can be raised by raising resistance, but that way, flow is also generally reduced. If it is necessary to raise pressure by raising flow or cardiac output, do this. There is nothing better than fluids. I think that Dr. Shoemaker's studies with blood and dextran, and various other agents, clearly illustrate that. But there comes a point at which fluids do not work for these patients. The earlier fluids and antibiotics are given to the patients in septic shock, the better. In this way, the stage of having to adjust resistance is never reached. And we hope that the same will be true in the earlier treatment of cardiogenic shock. That remains to be seen, but it has worked for other types of shock. Then, to increase *flow* as well as volume, the patient is given digitalis, of course. There are other drugs less commonly used, but digitalis is useful when the central venous pressure is high and there are hypotension and other signs of congestive failure. No single measurement is infallible. One has to coordinate all.

Now, how to adjust resistance: One of the simplest drugs to give is isoproterenol. I think a small dose is worth a trial for most patients, to see how they react to it. We have not found it good for a long-continued drip; but for quick resuscitation it is effective. It has theoretical attributes of the ideal drug: it raises cardiac output by direct effect and lowers resistance by dilating the voluntary muscle beds. But it has side-effects. After the patient has been given isoproterenol, and support of pressure is still needed and we want to get it by increasing flow, we turn to steroids as the most effective drug. Chlorpromazine, phenoxybenzamine, and phentolamine are other choices. If there still are problems, and a positive effect on the patient's heart is still needed to increase flow without increasing resistance, we may again try isoproterenol, epinephrine, or levarterenol for central inotropic effect. With this sort of plan I think that we can resuscitate almost all patients. Survival rate is about 60% because of other factors, such as late treatment of shock—abscesses not drained, various irremediable conditions, or other factors that we missed. However, by reviewing this plan one generally can decide when to use steroids and when to use other drugs or fluids.

Concluding Remarks

WESLEY W. SPINK, M.D.

First of all, on behalf of the participants I would like to thank the University of Illinois for their generosity and the courtesy to us. This has been a magnificent day. I have only one regret: that there were not more medical students and interns here. They are the persons who should hear controversy in medicine and hear that it is an empirical science, not always an exact science. As a matter of fact, there is a book, titled *Controversy in Internal Medicine*, which was published last year on this very subject. It is exciting to read, and a book that students should read. During the last 15 or 20 minutes I could not help thinking about poor Dr. Withering, who offered to the world almost 200 years ago, digitalis. I have recently reread his original monograph on how he used it, describing the manifestations of improvement and toxicity, and yet he had no idea how it worked.* When I was a medical student, not much was known about its action, and today we still lack some of the basic facts about digitalis. In discussing the steroids

---

* William Withering: *An Account of the Foxglove and Some of Its Medical Uses: With Practical Remarks on Dropsy; and Other Diseases.* Birmingham: Printed by M. Swinney, 207 pp. 1785.

today, we are in a somewhat analogous position concerning their use in shock. They have a variety of effects, but probably most important at the cellular level. They protect the integrity of the cell membrane. I look upon shock, no matter what the cause, as a dynamic mechanism, with anoxia the number one factor. This concept involves the inadequate perfusion of tissues by oxygenated blood. From then on, many processes are set in motion: the liberation of proteolytic enzymes, deterioration of metabolic cellular activity and, finally, death of the cell, even though adequate perfusion has been restored. I look upon shock as a form of "endogenous suicide" in which cellular death occurs with the liberation of proteolytic enzymes, and in which progressive and irreversible metabolic changes take place. It would seem to me that in the next few years much more attention should be paid to the metabolic effects of shock. What is happening to the host cells? We have a fairly good idea of what is happening hemodynamically. We need much more information of the metabolic factors involved in irreversible shock. That is why I think the steroids have such an important part in these studies. We have heard about a group of corticoids such as dexamethasone, cortisol and its analogues, but we haven't paid any attention to the mineralocorticoid, aldosterone. Now, it has been shown quite clearly in many experimental laboratories that aldosterone has effects similar to those of glucocorticoids, as far as shock is concerned. Why—we do not know. A large dose is deleterious and kills the animal. I would not recommend it for human use. I have very little else to add; I do not have a Cavanagh story. If I had one, I do not believe I would have the courage to tell it. But again I want to thank those who made this excellent symposium possible, Dr. Lloyd Nyhus, particularly Dr. Schumer, and Dr. Slayman.

Index